Top 65 Anti-inflammatory Superfoods

Diet for Life

Unlock Mediterranean Secrets to Longevity

Soothe Inflammation

Supercharge Your Immune System

Boost Heart, Joint, and Gut Health

Freeman Publishing

Contents

Introduction

There's an epidemic nobody is talking about and it's called Chronic Inflammation. Chronic inflammation can be defined as slow, long-term inflammation lasting several months to years. It most commonly manifests as arthritis, weakened immune systems, digestive issues, heart disorders, cancer, diabetes, or even transient, acute or chronic fatigue, and many people experience it on a day-to-day basis without even realizing it. These chronic inflammatory diseases are the most significant cause of death in the world, with 3 out of 5 people dying from chronic inflammatory diseases globally (Pahwa, Goyal, and Jialal 2023).

By understanding and addressing inflammation, you can help alleviate these burdens and improve your quality of life. This book aims to shed light on these health challenges, offering insights and solutions that are both practical and achievable. This book's purpose is to educate and inspire you. You will learn how an anti-inflammatory diet can transform your health. You will also discover the impact of superfoods and the Mediterranean diet on your body's natural defenses. These dietary changes hold the potential for long-term benefits, enhancing your vitality and longevity.

My name is Teri, and I have spent years exploring the intricate relationship between diet and well-being. My passion for helping others stems from personal experience and a deep commitment to uncovering the secrets of nutrition ever since my grandmother asked me to find her some Burdock Root tea to help the edema in her legs, caused by phlebitis. This was the 1970's, mind you, and there wasn't a health food store on every corner, especially not in the small town in Texas where I lived. I found the Burdock Root tea at a lovely little health food store in Lewisville Texas. The owner, who was very knowledgeable about every kind of herb and supplement, proceeded to educate me on all the benefits of eating healthy and using natural vitamins and herbs to support the immune system. I've been an advocate ever since and this book is driven by a personal desire to empower you to take control of your health through informed dietary choices. There are an array of choices you can make to break your bad food habits, and once you start feeling better, you will never look back.

DIET FOR LIFE is organized in clear, concise chapters, each focusing on a key aspect of inflammation and diet. We'll explore the digestive system, the power of antioxidants, and the role of nutrients like amino acids, vitamins, and minerals. You will find detailed explanations about how these elements work together to soothe inflammation and support your immune system. And, of course, included is an array of recipes—delicious, easy-to-make, Mediterranean-inspired dishes that make healthy eating a joy rather than a chore.

It is important to address common misconceptions. Anti-inflammatory diets are not about deprivation or strict rules. They are rather about making informed choices and taking small, sustainable steps. The results will not happen overnight, but with enough commitment, patience, and persistence, you will be rewarded. You will experience more energy, better digestion, and improved joint health.

I encourage you to actively engage with this book. Try out the recipes, follow the advice, and track your progress. Take notes, ask questions, and do not be afraid to experiment. Your involvement is critical, so by embracing the insights and strategies shared within these pages, you will uncover the secrets of well-being, longevity, and vitality.

Chapter 1

Understanding Inflammation and Gut Health

Have you ever wondered why you feel stiff in the morning or tired after a meal? These could be signs of inflammation, a term we hear often without understanding its full impact. Think of inflammation as your body's natural alarm system, designed to protect and heal. When you scrape your knee, inflammation rushes to the scene like a first responder. It is what causes swelling and redness, but it is also what kick-starts healing. However, when this alarm keeps ringing long after the threat has passed, it becomes a problem known as chronic inflammation, which wears down your body over time.

The Science of Inflammation: Causes and Effects

Inflammation is your body's built-in defense mechanism. When you catch a cold or twist an ankle, your body kicks into gear, sending immune cells to protect and repair (Pahwa, Goyal, and Jialal 2023). It starts rapidly, becomes severe in a short period, and symptoms may last for a few days (Pahwa, Goyal, and Jialal 2023). This process, known as acute inflammation, is vital. It is your body's way of saying, "I've got this" (Pahwa, Goyal, and Jialal 2023). The area gets warm and swollen as blood flow increases, bringing in nutrients and white blood cells to fight off invaders and begin repair work. You might notice pain, but that's your body's signal to take it easy, put a little ice on it and let the healing happen.

However, chronic inflammation is completely different. This type of inflammation persists over months or even years and can be very detrimental (Pahwa, Goyal, and Jialal 2023). Instead of healing, it starts to damage the body. Chronic inflammation can result from the following:

1. **Persistent Infection:** Pathogens like Mycobacterium tuberculosis, protozoa, and fungi that evade immune defenses and remain in tissues.
2. **Prolonged Irritant Exposure:** Non-degradable substances, such as silica dust and industrial chemicals, that resist breakdown.
3. **Autoimmune Disorders:** The immune system mistakenly attacks healthy tissue, causing diseases like RA (rheumatoid arthritis) and SLE (Systemic Lupus Erythematosus).
4. **Defective Inflammatory Response:** Dysfunctional immune cells leading to recurrent inflammation, as in auto-inflammatory disorders.
5. **Recurrent Acute Inflammation:** Repeated acute episodes or independent chronic conditions like tuberculosis and RA.
6. **Oxidative Stress and Mitochondrial Dysfunction:** Free radicals, AGEs (Advanced Glycation End products), uric acid crystals, and other

biochemical triggers driving inflammation (Pahwa, Goyal, and Jialal 2023).

However, and to many people's surprise, social, environmental, and lifestyle factors can be the source (Furman et al. 2019). **Poor dietary choices, like consuming processed foods high in sugar and unhealthy fats, often lead to inflammation** (Furman et al. 2019). These foods can trigger a cascade of inflammatory responses, disrupting normal bodily functions. **Environmental toxins, such as pollution and certain chemicals in household products, also play a role** (Furman et al. 2019). They can infiltrate your body, causing your immune system to react unnecessarily. Stress and lack of sleep further exacerbate the issue (Furman et al. 2019). **Chronic stress increases cortisol, a hormone that can promote inflammatory processes if elevated for too long** (Furman et al. 2019). Similarly, inadequate sleep does not give your body the time it needs to repair and reset, leaving you more susceptible to inflammation and setting up a cycle your body cannot escape.

The effects of chronic inflammation extend beyond the obvious. This is implicated in autoimmune disorders, where the body attacks its own tissues and even vital organs, such as the kidneys, mistaking them for foreign invaders (Kitscha 2021; Yaseen 2024). Conditions like rheumatoid arthritis and lupus are prime examples (Yaseen 2024). **Chronic inflammation is also a cause of heart disease, contributing to plaque buildup in arteries, which can lead to heart attacks and strokes** (Kitscha 2021). Persistent inflammation can also cause fatigue, mood swings, and even skin issues, making your day-to-day life harder than it needs to be.

Understanding the difference between beneficial and harmful inflammation is important. Beneficial inflammation is short-lived and necessary for healing. You will know it is helping when you notice initial pain and then swelling reducing over a few days. However, harmful inflammation lingers, often unnoticed, until significant damage occurs. Symptoms like constant fatigue, digestive problems, or unexplained aches might indicate chronic inflammation. Recognizing these signs early can prevent long-term damage and improve your well-being. You might find yourself waking up one morning, and the joints in your fingers are so stiff you cannot make a fist. I pinpointed MSG (monosodium glutamate) as the culprit after tracking my symptoms—every time I ate certain takeout or processed foods, I woke up with aching, stiff fingers. A bad flare-up followed a Chinese takeout dinner, confirming the pattern. Little old MSG, a frequent food additive that the doctors cannot agree on, but for me, it is the difference between fingers that bend and fingers that just ache. You will not believe the foods you are eating every day that contain MSG. Your doctor may not be able to tell you exactly why your joints ache more on a particular day, why you get those miserable headaches sometimes, or why a touchy stomach will occasionally keep you up all night. However, you can be your own food detective and figure out what you are sensitive to and how certain foods make you feel. Just do a quick Google search, you'll be surprised. You may even start reading labels more closely.

As this book explores the complexities of inflammation, remember that knowledge is your first defense. By recognizing the signs and understanding the causes, you are already taking a proactive step toward better health. This book will guide you through strategies to manage and reduce inflammation, helping you reclaim vitality and peace of mind.

The Gut-Inflammation Connection: How It Impacts Your Health

Your gut is an ecosystem that is home to trillions of bacteria that play an important role in your body's immune system. Located throughout the gastrointestinal tract is the gut-associated lymphoid tissue, or GALT, which acts as a central hub for immune response (Bemark et al. 2024). It is indispensable for the maintenance of gut homeostasis and overall human health (Bemark et al. 2024). When your gut is healthy, this system works efficiently, identifying threats and maintaining balance. However, when things go awry, inflammation can spread beyond the gut, affecting the entire body.

The connection between gut health and systemic inflammation is significant. **When the lining of the small and large intestines becomes compromised, it can lead to conditions like "leaky gut syndrome"** (Cleveland Clinic n.d.). Your gut lining acts as a sieve that normally lets through only nutrients and beneficial compounds, keeping toxins and pathogens out (Cleveland Clinic n.d.). But when this lining weakens, it becomes more like a leaky faucet, allowing harmful substances to enter the bloodstream. This triggers the immune system, resulting in widespread inflammation. Another issue is dysbiosis, an imbalance in the gut's bacterial and fungal microbiota (Hrncir 2022). When harmful bacteria outnumber the good, it can cause a chain reaction of inflammatory responses, impacting everything from digestion to mood. Has anyone ever told you to eat some yogurt after taking antibiotics? Well, they were on the right track to get your gut back in balance. You can get probiotics from delicious foods or supplements.

Our daily habits can significantly influence gut inflammation. A diet high in processed foods laden with additives and sugars can disrupt the delicate balance in your gut (Continental Hospitals Editorial Team 2023). White sugar and white flour are prime examples. These foods often lack the nutrients needed to support a healthy gut microbiome, leading to inflammation (Continental Hospitals Editorial Team 2023). The frequent use of antibiotics can also cause havoc. While these medications are sometimes necessary, they can indiscriminately kill both harmful and beneficial bacteria, leaving your gut microbiome out of balance, depleted, and vulnerable to inflammation. Stress and lack of sleep further complicate matters, as they can weaken your gut's ability to function properly, making inflammation even worse.

Fortunately, there are strategies to tackle gut-related inflammation. One of the most effective is incorporating anti-inflammatory foods into your diet. Replace highly processed foods that are full of salt, high fructose corn syrup, and chemical preservatives with less processed foods that contain no additives. Focus on whole, unprocessed foods rich in fiber, antioxidants, and healthy fats, such as fruits, leafy greens, nuts, and seeds. These foods nourish your gut and help reduce inflammation. Mindfulness practices can also play a significant role. Techniques like meditation and deep breathing exercises can lower stress (and cortisol) levels, improving gut health. When you manage stress effectively, your body can better regulate inflammation, leading to improved overall health (LeWine 2024).

To support your journey in understanding and improving gut health, I encourage you to keep a food and mood journal. This simple practice can help you identify patterns and triggers related to your diet and emotional well-being. Note what you eat, along with how you feel physically and mentally, and any symptoms you experience. I started keeping a small food notebook years ago when I was trying to lose weight before a wedding. It helped me keep track of my protein intake, held me accountable for snacking, and even helped me keep track of my water intake. Over time, you may notice correlations that can guide you in making informed dietary choices that support a healthy gut and reduce inflammation. Remember, small changes can lead to significant improvements in how you feel and function daily. Your gut plays a central role in your health, and by nurturing it, you can enhance your overall well-being.

The Digestive System: From Food to Nutrition

The digestive system is a marvel of biological engineering, transforming what we eat into the nutrients our bodies need. This intricate process begins the moment food enters your mouth. Chewing initiates digestion by breaking food into smaller pieces, making it easier for enzymes to go to work (National Institutes of Health n.d.). Saliva contains enzymes like amylase, which starts breaking down carbohydrates right there in your mouth (National Institutes of Health n.d.). As you swallow, the food travels down the esophagus, propelled by muscular contractions called peristalsis (National Institutes of Health n.d.). This process brings it to the stomach, where things heat up. The stomach produces hydrochloric acid and enzymes, such as pepsin, which further break down proteins (National Institutes of Health n.d.). This acidic environment helps kill bacteria and provides the ideal conditions for digestion to continue.

Once the partially digested food, now called chyme, leaves the stomach, it enters the small intestine—the real powerhouse of nutrient absorption (National Institutes of Health n.d.). Here, enzymes from the pancreas and bile from the liver mix with chyme to break down fats, carbohydrates, and proteins into their smallest components (National Institutes of Health n.d.). The small intestine, lined with tiny finger-like projections called villi, maximizes surface area, allowing for efficient nutrient absorption. These villi contain even smaller structures called microvilli, which absorb nutrients into the bloodstream. This stage is vital, as it is where vitamins, minerals, amino acids, and fatty acids are absorbed and transported to nourish every cell in your body (National Institutes of Health n.d.).

Each organ in the digestive system plays a major role. The stomach's production of acid aids in digestion and signals other digestive organs to start their processes. Proper nutrient absorption is important for reducing inflammation, as your body requires a steady supply of nutrients to maintain and repair tissues and to support immune function. However, if any part of this system falters, nutrient absorption can suffer. Malabsorption occurs when the small intestine cannot absorb nutrients effectively, leading to deficiencies that can affect your overall health (Sethi 2023). If your body cannot absorb fats, proteins, sugars, or vitamins, you may experience:

- **Fat Malabsorption:** Pale, foul-smelling, bulky stools that float or stick to the toilet.
- **Protein Malabsorption:** Dry hair, hair loss, or swelling (edema).
- **Sugar Malabsorption:** Bloating, gas, or explosive diarrhea.
- **Vitamin malabsorption:** Anemia, malnutrition, low blood pressure, weight loss, or muscle wasting (Sethi 2023).

Several factors can disrupt digestion. Stress, for instance, diverts energy away from the digestive system, slowing down processes and potentially leading to issues like indigestion and bloating. Similarly, dehydration can impair digestion, as water is critical for producing digestive juices and facilitating the movement of food through the digestive tract. Without adequate hydration, digestion can become sluggish, leading to constipation and discomfort. I was once told to drink a glass of water 20 to 30 minutes before a meal or snack in order to maximize hydration without diluting digestive enzymes, and I have followed this routine ever since. This practice also helps ensure I get in my 2 liters of water every day.

Understanding these processes highlights the importance of nurturing your digestive system. By recognizing the role of each part, from enzymes to organs, and the importance of nutrient absorption, you can make informed decisions about your diet and lifestyle. Stress management and staying hydrated are as important as choosing the right foods. The digestive system is the gateway to your health, and by caring for it, you lay the foundation for your overall well-being.

The Role of the Microbiome: Tiny Microorganisms in the Gut

Your microbiome is a diverse community of trillions of microorganisms teeming with life and activity that call your gut home. These tiny residents, including bacteria, fungi, and viruses, live in harmony with your body, forming a symbiotic relationship that is critical for your health (Belkaid and Hand 2015). They each play a key role in maintaining balance and supporting human physiology (Belkaid and Hand 2015). While bacteria are the most abundant and studied, fungi and viruses also contribute to this complex ecosystem (Belkaid and Hand 2015). They work together to aid digestion, synthesize essential vitamins, and, most importantly, support your immune system in keeping inflammation at bay.

Your microbiome's influence on inflammation is significant. Beneficial bacteria regulate immune responses and prevent unnecessary inflammatory reactions. They produce short-chain fatty acids, such as butyrate, which have anti-inflammatory properties (Shin et al. 2023). These fatty acids serve as fuel for the cells lining your gut, strengthening the critical barrier that keeps harmful substances out. A well-fed gut lining means less chance for inflammation to take root and spread (Shin et al. 2023). When the microbiome is balanced, it acts as a vigilant gatekeeper, ensuring that inflammation is kept in check. However, when the balance tips, things can quickly go awry, leading to a cascade of inflammatory responses.

Our everyday choices have a big impact on the health of our microbiome. Diet, for instance, plays a major role in either supporting or disrupting these microbial communities. A high-fiber diet, rich in fruits, vegetables, and whole grains, provides the nourishment that beneficial bacteria thrive on (Lewis 2024). Fiber acts as a prebiotic, feeding the good bacteria and promoting their growth (Lewis 2024). On the other hand, a diet low in fiber and high in processed foods can starve these helpful microbes, allowing harmful ones to flourish. Incorporating probiotics, found in foods like yogurt, kefir and sauerkraut, can also improve your microbiome (Lewis 2024). These live beneficial bacteria can help restore balance and support your gut health (Lewis 2024).

When the microbiome is out of balance, the consequences can be far-reaching. An imbalance, often referred to as dysbiosis, can lead to an increased risk of inflammatory diseases (Belkaid and Hand 2015). Conditions like type 2 diabetes, obesity, and inflammatory bowel disease have been linked to an unhealthy microbiome (Belkaid and Hand 2015). When harmful bacteria outnumber the beneficial ones, they can trigger inflammatory pathways, contributing to these chronic conditions. Moreover, an imbalanced microbiome can weaken your immune system, making you more susceptible to general infections and illnesses.

It is extremely important to be mindful of lifestyle habits to maintain a healthy gut microbiome. Consuming a variety of whole, unprocessed foods, especially those high in fiber, is a key strategy. Additionally, reducing stress, staying hydrated, and getting adequate sleep all contribute to a thriving microbiome. These practices help create an environment where beneficial microbes can flourish, keeping inflammation in check and supporting your overall health. By nurturing your microbiome, you are enhancing your body's ability to defend against inflammation and disease. Remember, these tiny gut microorganisms are integral to your health, and by promoting their growth, you are investing in a healthier, more resilient you.

Symptoms and Diagnosis: Recognizing Signs of Gut Issues

Gut issues often manifest through a host of uncomfortable symptoms. Bloating and gas are among the most common indicators that something might be amiss in your digestive tract. Abdominal pain is another frequent complaint, varying from a dull ache to sharp, cramping sensations that can leave you doubled over. These symptoms are your body's way of signaling that the digestive system isn't functioning optimally, possibly due to food sensitivities, inflammation, or other underlying issues. Understanding these signs is vital for your food detective project, as they can provide valuable clues about what is happening inside your gut.

When these symptoms persist and become disruptive, it is important to seek a proper diagnosis to uncover the root cause and address it effectively. One of the primary tools for diagnosing gut issues is an endoscopy. This procedure involves inserting a thin, flexible tube with a camera into the digestive tract, allowing doctors to visually inspect the esophagus, stomach, and small intestine (John Hopkins Medicine n.d.). An endoscopy can help identify conditions like ulcers, inflammation, or structural abnormalities that might be contributing to your symptoms. Stool analysis is another valuable diagnostic tool, providing insights into the microbial composition of your gut (John Hopkins Medicine n.d.). By examining a stool sample, healthcare professionals can detect infections, inflammation, and other abnormalities in the digestive system. These diagnostic methods, while sometimes daunting, can offer clarity and direction, helping to formulate a targeted treatment plan.

Early detection of gut issues is paramount. Left unaddressed, these problems can escalate into chronic health conditions that are much more difficult to manage. Ignoring persistent gut symptoms can result in long-term damage, affecting not only the digestive system but also overall health and well-being. **Chronic inflammation in the gut has been linked to a range of serious conditions, including autoimmune disorders and even certain cancers** (Furman et al. 2019). By paying attention to your body's signals and seeking medical evaluation early on, you can prevent these more severe outcomes and maintain better health over the long term.

Knowing when to consult a healthcare professional is an important part of managing your health effectively. If you experience persistent symptoms like bloating, gas, or abdominal pain that interfere with your daily life, it is time to seek medical advice. Start by discussing your symptoms with a primary care provider, who can perform an initial assessment and recommend further testing if needed. It may be helpful to keep a symptom diary, noting when discomfort occurs, what you have eaten, and any other relevant factors. This information can provide valuable context for your healthcare provider, aiding in diagnosis and treatment planning. If your primary doctor suspects a more complex issue, they might refer you to a gastroenterologist, a specialist in digestive health who can offer more in-depth evaluation and management options. Remember, seeking help is a proactive step in taking control of your health, and it is a good idea to ask for professional guidance when your body is sending signals that something is not right.

Common Gut Disorders: IBS, Celiac, and More

Two of the most common gut conditions people face are Irritable Bowel Syndrome (IBS) and Celiac Disease (Verdu, Armstrong, and Murray 2009). IBS is a bit of a mystery, affecting up to 10% of the American population and causing symptoms like abdominal pain, bloating, and altered bowel habits (Verdu, Armstrong, and Murray 2009). It is a functional disorder, meaning the gut looks normal but does not work as it should (Verdu, Armstrong, and Murray 2009). Stress, diet, and gut-brain interactions play a significant role in triggering symptoms. On the other hand, Celiac Disease is an autoimmune disorder where ingesting gluten triggers an immune response that damages the small intestine's lining (Verdu, Armstrong, and Murray 2009). Gluten is a protein found in wheat, barley and rye. It is a complex mixture of proteins, primarily gliadin and glutenin, that gives dough its elasticity and bread its texture. This immune response reaction can lead to nutrient malabsorption, fatigue, and a host of other symptoms if left unchecked (Verdu, Armstrong, and Murray 2009).

The causes of these disorders are complex. IBS does not have a clear-cut cause but is thought to result from a combination of genetic, environmental, and psychological factors (Verdu,

Armstrong, and Murray 2009). Triggers often include certain foods, stress, and hormonal changes. Celiac Disease, however, has a strong genetic component. It requires the presence of specific genes and the consumption of gluten, found in wheat, barley, rye, triticale, and some wheat varieties like spelt, durum, and farro, as well as in some processed foods and snacks, to activate the disease (Verdu, Armstrong, and Murray 2009). Environmental factors, like gut infections and changes in gut microbiota, may also influence its development. Gluten intolerance, distinct from Celiac Disease, can cause similar symptoms but without the autoimmune response, making it more difficult to diagnose.

Managing these conditions requires a tailored approach. For IBS, the Low-FODMAP diet has gained traction as an effective management strategy (Magge and Lembo 2012). FODMAP stands for fermentable oligosaccharides, disaccharides, monosaccharides, and polyols, which are short-chain carbohydrates (sugars) that the small intestines absorb poorly (Magge and Lembo 2012). These fermentable carbohydrates can exacerbate IBS symptoms by increasing gas and water in the intestines (Magge and Lembo 2012). By identifying and reducing foods high in FODMAPs, such as certain fruits, vegetables, and dairy products, many people find relief. It is a diet best undertaken with the guidance of a dietitian to ensure balanced nutrition. For those with Celiac Disease, a strict gluten-free diet is the only treatment. This means eliminating all sources of gluten from the diet to prevent immune responses and intestinal damage (Verdu, Armstrong, and Murray 2009). It can be challenging, given gluten's prevalence in many foods, but with careful planning and vigilance, individuals can live symptom-free.

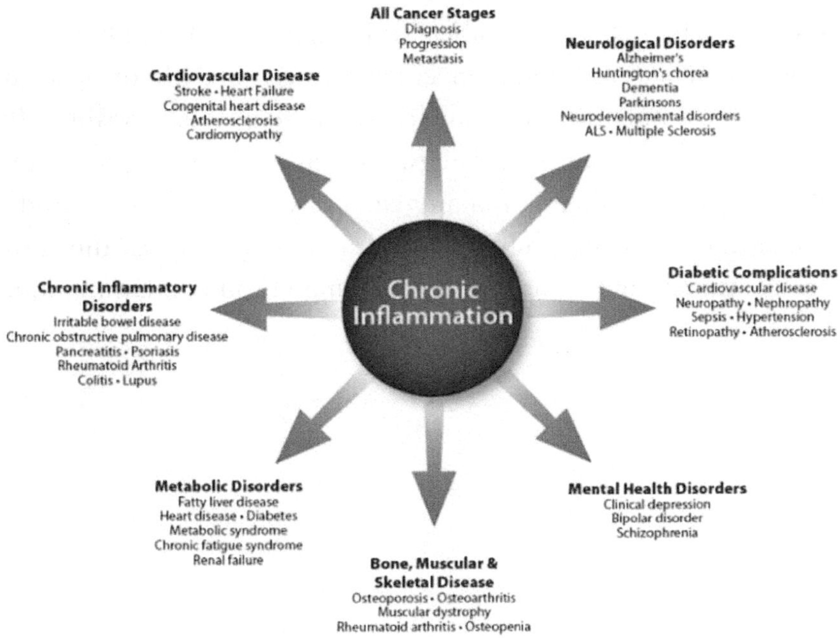

A personalized approach is important in managing these disorders. Each person's triggers and responses can vary, making it important to work closely with healthcare providers. A gastroenterologist can help diagnose and monitor the condition, while a dietitian can tailor dietary strategies that suit individual needs. Keeping a food diary can be immensely helpful in identifying specific triggers and tracking symptoms. Lifestyle modifications, such as stress management techniques and regular exercise, can also complement dietary changes and further improve quality of life.

Living with gut disorders does not have to be a constant uphill battle. With the right knowledge and tools, you can overcome these challenges more effectively. Understanding your body, recognizing triggers, and working with healthcare professionals will allow you to take control. The goal is to find a balance that allows you to live comfortably and enjoyably. Though it may require patience and persistence, achieving a life where your gut health does not dictate your daily activities is possible. By embracing a personalized strategy, you can reduce symptoms and enhance your well-being, making each day a little brighter and a lot healthier. The next chapter of this book discusses the most effective nutritional means for minimizing chronic inflammation.

Chapter 2

Nutritional Foundations for Reducing Inflammation

Have you ever noticed how a freshly peeled apple quickly turns brown when it comes in contact with air? This simple transformation is a visible reminder of oxidation, a process happening in our bodies daily. While oxidation is natural, excessive free radicals— atoms or groups of atoms that have a single unpaired electron—which are the byproducts of oxidation, can lead to cellular damage and inflammation (Lobo et al. 2010). This is where antioxidants come into play. They are the heroes that neutralize these free radicals, acting as a shield against cellular damage (Lobo et al. 2010). Just like the natural antioxidant, citric acid, in lemon juice applied to your apple slices keeps them from turning brown for that yummy fruit salad, antioxidants come to the rescue in many forms. Free radicals in our food are one of the biggest causes of internal damage. A major source of free radicals is fried foods where the oil has been heated beyond its smoke point. Reactive oxygen species (ROS), a type of free radical, are particularly notorious for contributing to chronic inflammation when left unchecked (Lobo et al. 2010). Here, antioxidants work to neutralize ROS, preventing them from wreaking havoc on your cells (Lobo et al. 2010).

Antioxidants: Fighting Against Inflammation

Antioxidants are abundant in a variety of foods, particularly in blueberries, blackberries, cranberries, raspberries, and strawberries. These fruits are packed with nutrients that support your body's natural defenses. Blueberries, for instance, contain anthocyanins, powerful compounds known for their antioxidant properties (Ashique et al. 2024). These substances counteract oxidative stress by neutralizing free radicals, decreasing the likelihood of developing chronic illnesses such as cardiovascular disease, cancer, and neurological disorders (Ashique et al. 2024). Strawberries provide vitamin C, another potent antioxidant. Dark chocolate and green tea also deserve a spot on your plate. Dark chocolate, when enjoyed in moderation, offers flavonoids that help reduce inflammation. Green tea, rich in catechins, is a soothing beverage that supports heart and brain health while combating oxidative stress. Including these foods in your diet can enhance your antioxidant intake, giving your body the ability to fight inflammation.

The connection between antioxidants and reduced inflammation is important. When antioxidants neutralize free radicals, they reduce oxidative stress—a key player in inflammation (Lobo et al. 2010). Oxidative stress occurs when the balance between free radicals and antioxidants tips in favor of the former, leading to damage at the cellular level (Lobo et al. 2010). This damage can trigger inflammatory pathways, making it harder for your body to repair and heal (Lobo et al. 2010). By reducing oxidative stress, antioxidants help lower inflammation, supporting better health outcomes (Lobo et al. 2010). This reduction in inflammation can lead to improved joint health, enhanced immune function, and even a lower risk of chronic diseases like heart disease and cancer.

Incorporating more antioxidants into your daily meals does not have to be a chore. Simple changes can make a significant difference. Start by adding a handful of berries to your breakfast cereal or yogurt. One of my go-to breakfasts is steel-cut Irish oatmeal with berries or dark chocolate mini chips and some chopped almonds or walnuts. Delicious and very filling. Consider swapping your usual morning coffee for a cup of green tea, giving you a gentle caffeine boost while flooding your system with antioxidants. I drink 3 to 4 cups of organic green tea every day, so I opt for decaffeinated tea. Experiment with dark chocolate as a dessert option with your favorite berries. Just a small square, at least 70% cocoa, can satisfy your sweet tooth and offer health benefits. Also, do not overlook the power of herbs and spices like turmeric and cinnamon. Sprinkle cinnamon on your oatmeal or add turmeric to your soups and stews for a tasty antioxidant boost. These small tweaks can elevate your diet and help to keep inflammation at bay.

Interactive Element: Suggestions for Adding Antioxidants into your Meals

Consider planning your meals around antioxidant-rich foods to support your overall health. Aim to include at least one meal or snack per day that features ingredients like berries, dark chocolate, green tea, or antioxidant-packed spices. Write down your meal plan and track how you feel throughout the week. Do you notice changes in your energy levels or mood? This simple exercise can help you recognize the benefits of increasing your antioxidant intake and make these nutrient-dense foods a regular part of your diet.

For breakfast, choose a whole grain base such as oatmeal, homemade granola, muesli, cracked farro, quinoa, or amaranth. Top it with fresh berries or dried cranberries for a burst of antioxidants. Add some almonds, walnuts, chia seeds, hemp seeds, sunflower seeds, or pumpkin seeds for extra texture and nutrients. Muesli, an uncooked grain mix, can be enjoyed hot or cold. Try adding ¼ cup of muesli to Greek yogurt for a calcium-rich, protein-packed breakfast. To mix things up, instead of oatmeal every day, soak your muesli overnight in rice or soy milk for a creamy, no-cook option, or cook it on the stovetop with water for a warm and satisfying meal. Finish with your favorite fresh berries for natural sweetness and extra nutrients.

Muesli and granola contain similar ingredients—oats or other grains, nuts, seeds, and dried fruit. The key difference is that granola is baked with a sweetener like honey or brown sugar for a crunchier texture. You can reduce carbohydrates by swapping out some grains for coconut flakes. Making granola at home lets you control the sugar content and avoid the high levels found in many store-bought varieties. A standard serving is about ¼ cup, perfect for sprinkling over Greek yogurt for a dessert-like breakfast. Save time by preparing granola and muesli in one batch. Start with 2–3 cups of rolled oats. Before baking, set aside a portion for muesli. To make granola, mix in a healthy oil and natural sweetener, then add your favorite nuts, seeds, and dried fruit. Spread the mixture in a single layer on a baking sheet and bake at 325°F for about 30 minutes, stirring occasionally for even crispness. Keep ¼ cup portions ready to go for a quick snack.

Flaxseed is a powerful superfood, but to get the most nutrients, it needs to be freshly ground. Once ground, flaxseed quickly loses its nutritional value due to oxidation and exposure to heat and light. Use a coffee grinder to grind fresh flax seeds and add them to your smoothie, oatmeal, or muesli for a nutritional boost. By incorporating these antioxidant-rich foods into your daily routine, you'll not only enjoy delicious meals but also support your overall well-being, and I guarantee you won't feel as hungry or have that sugar crash that usually follows processed food snacks.

Phytochemicals: Nature's Defense Against Inflammation

Phytochemicals are fascinating compounds found in plants, acting as natural barriers against inflammation. These bioactive substances are not just responsible for the colors, flavors, and aromas of fruits and vegetables, but they also offer a plethora of health benefits (Kumar et al. 2023). Two key types of phytochemicals that play a significant role in managing inflammation are flavonoids and carotenoids (Han, Zhang, and Skibsted 2012). Flavonoids, found in a variety of fruits, vegetables, teas, and wines, are known for their antioxidant and anti-inflammatory properties. They help to protect cells from damage and reduce inflammation by inhibiting the pathways that trigger inflammatory responses (Han, Zhang, and Skibsted 2012). Carotenoids, on the other hand, are the pigments that give carrots, sweet potatoes, and pumpkins their orange hue. These compounds are powerful antioxidants that help to prevent oxidative damage and support immune function (Han, Zhang, and Skibsted 2012). By including a variety of these delicious, colorful plant foods in your diet, you can benefit from these protective compounds and support your body's natural defenses against inflammation.

The anti-inflammatory properties of phytochemicals are remarkable. They work by inhibiting inflammatory pathways, which are the biochemical routes through which inflammation is triggered and sustained in the body. By blocking these pathways, phytochemicals can help to reduce the production of inflammatory markers and prevent chronic inflammation from taking hold. This makes them a useful tool in managing conditions associated with inflammation, such as arthritis, heart disease, and diabetes (Kumar et al. 2023). In addition to their direct anti-inflammatory effects, phytochemicals also support overall health by enhancing immune function, improving gut health, regulating gene transcription, and providing protection against lung and prostate cancers (Kumar et al. 2023). By incorporating a diverse range of phytochemical-rich foods into your diet, you can help protect your body from the harmful effects of inflammation and promote long-term health.

Foods rich in phytochemicals should be staples in your kitchen. Cruciferous vegetables like broccoli and kale are excellent sources of these compounds, particularly glucosinolates, which have been studied for their cancer-fighting properties, lowering the risk of lung and colorectal cancers in some epidemiological studies (Higdon et al. 2007). These vegetables are packed with vitamins and minerals and also offer powerful anti-inflammatory effects. Citrus fruits, such as oranges and grapefruits, are also rich in flavonoids and vitamin C, which can help reduce inflammation and support immune health. Make sure that you do not overlook the power of herbs and spices, either. Many of these contain phytochemicals that can enhance the flavor of your meals while providing additional health benefits. Add a variety of these foods to your diet to enjoy their delicious flavors while reaping the rewards of their anti-inflammatory properties.

Incorporating phytochemical-rich foods into your daily meals is easier than you might think. One delicious way to do this is by blending leafy greens like spinach or kale into your morning smoothie. This will boost your intake of fiber and nutrients and also provide a hefty dose of anti-inflammatory phytochemicals. You can also experiment with creating your own salad dressings made from fresh citrus juice, which adds a zesty kick while delivering a burst of flavonoids and don't include sugar or MSG. Try using a variety of vegetables in your salads and stir-fries to create colorful, nutrient-dense dishes that are as pleasing to the eye as they are to the palate. By making these simple adjustments to your meals, you can enhance your diet with the power of phytochemicals, keeping inflammation at bay in the most delicious way.

Amino Acids and Proteins: Building Blocks for Health

Proteins and amino acids are critical for maintaining the structure and function of our bodies (Kubala 2025). Proteins are made up of amino acids, which are often referred to as the building blocks of life (Kubala 2025). They repair tissues, build muscle, and produce enzymes and hormones. There are 20 amino acids in total, but our bodies can only produce 11 of them naturally (Kubala 2025). The remaining nine, known as essential amino acids, must come from our diet (Kubala 2025). This makes it crucial to consume a variety of foods to get all the amino acids needed for optimal health.

The nine amino acids we want to make sure are present in our daily diet are:

- Histidine
- Isoleucine
- Leucine
- Lysine

- Methionine
- Phenylalanine
- Threonine
- Tryptophan
- Valine (Kubala 2025).

Sources of the complete proteins that contain all nine essential amino acids include beef, chicken, turkey, pork, fish, eggs, milk, yogurt, cheese, soy products like tofu and edamame, quinoa, and buckwheat (Kubala 2025). Incomplete proteins lack some essential amino acids and include nuts and seeds, rice, wheat, corn, beans, and lentils (Kubala 2025).

In anti-inflammatory diets, certain protein sources stand out, but in a good way. Fatty fish such as salmon are rich in omega-3 fatty acids and are known for their anti-inflammatory properties, thus making them a top choice (Spritzler 2023). These fatty acids can help reduce inflammation, support heart health, and improve brain function (Spritzler 2023). Legumes and beans, such as lentils and chickpeas, are excellent plant-based protein sources that also offer fiber and antioxidants. They work wonders in reducing inflammation due to their nutrient-dense profile. Incorporating these proteins into your diet can provide the necessary fuel for your body while keeping inflammation at bay.

Protein plays an interesting role in gut health. The type and amount of protein you consume can influence your gut microbiota, the community of microbes living in your digestive tract. A balanced intake supports the growth of beneficial bacteria, which can help reduce inflammation and improve digestive health. However, an excess of animal proteins, particularly from red and processed meats, can negatively affect gut health by promoting the growth of harmful bacteria. To support a healthy gut, focus on a mix of plant and animal proteins, guaranteeing a diverse and balanced diet.

Finding the right balance of protein intake is important. Combining different plant proteins, such as beans, lentils, and whole grains, can provide a complete amino acid profile similar to that of animal proteins. This is especially important for those following a vegetarian or vegan diet. For those who eat animal proteins, practicing portion control is necessary to avoid potential negative effects on gut health and inflammation. For those of you who cannot pass up a high-quality steak once in a while, be aware that 3 ounces is considered an acceptable portion size. Add quinoa and a serving of spinach, broccoli, or asparagus as a side for a varied diet that includes both plant and animal proteins, ensuring you get the benefits of both without overloading on any one source. This balance supports muscle, tissue, and gut health.

Vitamins and Minerals: Essentials for a Balanced Diet

When it comes to reducing inflammation, vitamins and minerals are most effective. In particular, vitamin D, magnesium, and zinc stand out for their significant anti-inflammatory effects. Vitamin D helps regulate the immune system, which reduces chronic inflammation. Fatty fish, such as salmon and mackerel, and egg yolks are optimal sources of this indispensable vitamin. Additionally, fortified foods like certain dairy products and cereals can help you get your daily dose. Magnesium plays a vital role in over 300 biochemical reactions in your body and is known for calming inflammation. You can find it in nuts, seeds, and leafy greens. If you need a magnesium supplement, some people like a combination of magnesium glycinate and magnesium malate. Personally, I take magnesium L-threonate capsules at bedtime to help me sleep. Zinc, another inflammation fighter, is needed for immune function. It can be found in foods like pumpkin seeds, lentils, and chickpeas. These minerals do not just work in isolation, but rather, they support each other, creating a robust defense against inflammation.

Vitamins and minerals also support immune function. They promote the production and activity of white blood cells, which are your body's frontline defense against pathogens. Vitamin D, for instance, enhances the pathogen-fighting effects of monocytes and macrophages—white blood cells that are vital parts of immune defense. Magnesium helps maintain a healthy immune response level, ensuring that it does not go into overdrive and cause unnecessary inflammation. Zinc is known for its role in developing and activating T-lymphocytes, which are necessary for adaptive immunity. With these nutrients, your immune system can function efficiently, reducing the risk of chronic inflammation and related health problems.

To make sure that you are getting enough of these essential nutrients, it is important to incorporate a variety of rich food sources into your diet. If you find it challenging to get these nutrients through food alone, consider using fortified products. Many cereals and plant-based milk alternatives are fortified with vitamin D and other important nutrients, making it easier to meet your daily needs. Just be sure any processed foods you choose are not loaded with salt, sugar, or unhealthy fats. Look for quality, less-processed foods. Including a range of these foods in your diet will help you maintain a balanced intake of these important nutrients.

Daily habits can make a big difference in guaranteeing that you get enough vitamins and minerals. Start by planning meals that incorporate nutrient-dense foods. For breakfast, try an omelet with spinach and mushrooms or oatmeal topped with nuts and seeds. If you are concerned about fat or cholesterol, opt for an egg white omelet. Lunch might be a salad featuring leafy greens, avocado, and grilled chicken or fish. For dinner, enjoy a piece of salmon with quinoa and roasted vegetables. These meals are delicious and also packed with the vitamins and minerals your body needs to combat inflammation. Whole grains are also a great source of magnesium and can be easily incorporated into meals. Use brown rice, quinoa, or ancient-grain pasta as a base for your dishes. These simple adjustments in your eating patterns can significantly boost your nutrient intake, supporting both your immune system and your efforts to reduce inflammation.

The Fiber Factor: Types and Benefits for Gut Health

Fiber works to keep your digestive system running smoothly. There are two main types of dietary fiber: soluble and insoluble (Mayo Clinic Staff 2024). Soluble fiber dissolves in water to form a gel-like substance in the stomach, which can help lower blood cholesterol and glucose levels (Mayo Clinic Staff 2024). You will find it in foods like oats, apples, beans, and legumes (Mayo Clinic Staff 2024). Insoluble fiber, on the other hand, does not dissolve in water. It adds bulk to the stool and helps food pass more quickly through the stomach and intestines, which is necessary for regular digestion (Mayo Clinic Staff 2024). Sources include whole grains and vegetables. Both types of fiber play a role in promoting better health, but they do it in slightly different ways.

Fiber supports digestive health by acting as a prebiotic, which means it feeds the good bacteria in your gut. This is vital because these bacteria help keep your digestive system healthy and reduce inflammation. When you consume fiber, it encourages the growth of beneficial bacteria, enhancing the diversity of your gut microbiome. A diverse microbiome is associated with better health outcomes, including reduced inflammation and improved digestion. Fiber also helps regulate bowel movements, prevent constipation, and support overall digestive health. By keeping things moving smoothly, fiber reduces the risk of developing diverticulitis, a condition where small, bulging pouches form in the digestive tract (Mayo Clinic Staff 2024). This makes fiber important in maintaining a healthy gut.

Incorporating fiber-rich foods into your diet is easier than you might think. Start with whole grains, such as brown rice, quinoa, and Essene or Ezekiel bread, which provide a hearty dose of insoluble fiber. Vegetables like broccoli, carrots, and brussels sprouts are also excellent options. When it comes to fruits, keep the skin on whenever possible, as it contains a significant amount of fiber. Apples, pears, and berries are great examples. Legumes, including beans, lentils, and chickpeas, are another fantastic source of fiber and can be added to soups, stews, or salads. By choosing a variety of these foods, you can easily meet your daily fiber needs and support your anti-inflammatory diet.

If you are new to eating a high-fiber diet, it is important to increase your intake gradually to avoid digestive discomfort. Start by adding small amounts of fiber-rich foods to your meals and gradually increase the quantity over time. This allows your digestive system to adjust and helps prevent bloating and gas. Additionally, make sure to drink plenty of water, as fiber works best when it absorbs water, making your stool softer and easier to pass. Aim for at least 2 liters of water a day to keep things moving smoothly. Consider spreading your fiber intake throughout the day rather than consuming a large amount in one sitting. By taking these steps, you can enjoy the benefits of fiber without experiencing any discomfort.

Micronutrients: Small but Important Inflammation Fighters

Micronutrients may sound like a small detail in the grand scheme of nutrition, but their impact on your health is anything but minor. These are the vitamins and minerals that your body requires in small amounts, yet they play significant roles in maintaining health and reducing inflammation. Selenium, for example, is a powerful antioxidant that helps protect your cells from damage (Huang, Rose, and Hoffmann 2012). It supports the immune system and prevents chronic inflammation by neutralizing free radicals (Huang, Rose, and Hoffmann 2012). A deficiency in selenium can leave your body vulnerable, increasing the risk of inflammation-related diseases.

To keep these inflammation fighters in your diet, focus on foods rich in micronutrients. Brazil nuts are a standout choice for selenium. Eating just two Brazil nuts can provide your daily requirement, making them a convenient and tasty option. Leafy greens, like spinach and kale, are packed with numerous vitamins and minerals, including vitamin K, which plays a role in reducing inflammation. Whole grains, such as quinoa and brown rice, offer a variety of micronutrients that support overall health, from magnesium to B vitamins. By including these nutrient-dense foods in your meals, you ensure a steady supply of vital nutrients that help reduce inflammation.

RECAP: A lack of certain micronutrients can exacerbate inflammation and contribute to chronic diseases. When your body does not get enough of these critical nutrients, it struggles to perform essential functions, leaving you more susceptible to conditions like heart disease, diabetes, and autoimmune disorders. For instance, low levels of selenium or magnesium can impair your body's ability to manage inflammation. Addressing these deficiencies through diet can significantly reduce your risk of developing diseases. It is a reminder that even small dietary changes can have a big impact on health.

Maintaining a balance of micronutrients in your diet requires a thoughtful approach. Start by embracing a diverse diet that includes a wide variety of foods. This ensures you get a broad spectrum of vitamins and minerals, each contributing its unique benefits. Plan your meals with variety in mind, rotating different fruits, vegetables, grains, and proteins throughout the week. This keeps your meals interesting and helps you avoid any nutrient gaps. Consider using a meal planner or keeping a food journal to track your intake and ensure you are meeting your nutritional needs. If you suspect you might be lacking in certain micronutrients, consult with a healthcare provider who can recommend dietary changes or supplements as needed.

As you continue exploring the nutritional foundations that support your well-being, remember that even small adjustments can lead to significant improvements in how you feel and function. This understanding of micronutrients completes our exploration of the nutritional elements that can help reduce inflammation. The following chapter discusses the top 65 anti-inflammatory foods and their importance.

Chapter 3

Top 65 Anti-inflammatory Superfoods

Chronic inflammation is linked to various health issues, including heart disease and diabetes. Fortunately, certain foods help combat inflammation and promote overall well-being. This chapter highlights 65 powerful anti-inflammatory superfoods that support optimal health. From antioxidant-rich blueberries to omega-3-packed salmon, each food on this list offers unique benefits. Whether boosting your diet with fiber, healthy fats, or important nutrients, these superfoods provide a natural way to strengthen your body's defenses.

Top Anti-Inflammatory Superfoods

Here is my self-created list of the 65+ Top Anti-Inflammatory Superfoods you should incorporate as often as possible:

- **Blueberries**
- **Avocado**
- **Olive Oil**
- **Oatmeal**

- **Green Tea, herbal teas**
- **Mushrooms**
- **Fish:** Salmon, sardines, tuna, sea bass, trout, herring, mackerel, shellfish
- **Whole grains:** Quinoa, farro, amaranth
- **Nuts:** Walnuts, almonds, pecans, Brazil nuts, pine nuts, pistachios
- **Berries:** Blackberries, raspberries, strawberries, cranberries, acai, goji
- **Dark leafy greens:** Kale, spinach, arugula, Swiss chard, collard, turnip greens
- **Legumes:** Edamame, beans, lentils, peas
- **Seeds:** Chia seeds, flax seeds, hemp seeds, sunflower seeds, pumpkin seeds
- **Fruit:** Cherries, grapes, pears, apples, grapefruit, pomegranates, kiwi, dates, figs, mango, guava, papaya, passion fruit, watermelon, dragon fruit, jackfruit
- **Cruciferous vegetables:** Broccoli, cauliflower, brussels sprouts
- **Root vegetables:** Carrots, beets
- **Tofu**
- **Sweet potatoes**
- **Dark chocolate**
- **Garlic**
- **Ginger**
- **Turmeric**
- **Eggs**
- **Greek yogurt**
- **Coconut**
- **Tomatoes**
- **BONUS SUPERFOOD (My Favorite! Pomegranate seeds !** Sprinkle on a salad or salmon filet. Top off greek yogurt or add to a smoothie or fruit

salad. Colorful little flavor bombs that dress up almost anything. Yum !

Blueberries: An Anti-inflammatory Necessity

At first glance, blueberries might seem like any other berry, but their benefits are far-reaching and well-documented. Blueberries are one of nature's most potent sources of antioxidants, particularly anthocyanins, which lend them their deep blue hue (Kalt et al. 2019). These phytochemicals work tirelessly to combat free radicals, and when consumed regularly, blueberries can reduce the risk of cardiovascular disease and type 2 diabetes (Kalt et al. 2019). Studies have shown that regular consumption of blueberries can lead to a reduction in C-reactive protein levels, a marker of inflammation (Kalt et al. 2019). This is significant because high levels of C-reactive protein are linked to an increased risk of chronic diseases, including heart disease and diabetes. Blueberries also have a positive effect on vascular health, improving blood flow and reducing blood pressure.By integrating blueberries into your diet, you are both indulging in their delicious taste and actively protecting your health.

The nutritional profile of blueberries is impressive. They are packed with Vitamin C and Vitamin K, essential nutrients that support immune function and bone health, respectively. Vitamin C is well-known for its role in boosting the immune system and protecting against infections. Meanwhile, Vitamin K is critical for blood clotting and maintaining healthy bones. Blueberries are also a good source of dietary fiber, which aids in digestion and helps keep you feeling full longer. This combination of vitamins, minerals, and fiber makes blueberries a nutritional powerhouse.

Incorporating blueberries into your daily routine is both easy and enjoyable. One of the simplest ways is by adding them to your morning smoothie or yogurt parfait. Their sweet-tart flavor pairs wonderfully with creamy Greek yogurt, creating a delicious and nutritious breakfast or snack. You can also sprinkle them over your oatmeal or cereal for an antioxidant boost. If you are feeling adventurous, you might try tossing a handful of blueberries into your salads for a burst of color and flavor.

Recipe for a Blueberry Smoothie

Try this simple blueberry smoothie recipe to kickstart your day with a dose of antioxidants. Blend 1 cup of fresh or frozen blueberries with one banana, 1 cup of almond milk, and a tablespoon of fresh ground flaxseeds. Add a handful of spinach and a tablespoon of chia seeds for extra oomph. Blend until smooth and enjoy a refreshing smoothie that is packed with nutrients that support your health goals.

Salmon: Omega-3 Rich Superfood

When it comes to reducing inflammation and promoting heart health, salmon stands out as a true superfood due to its rich content of omega-3 fatty acids. These vital fats, primarily EPA (eicosapentaenoic acid) and DHA (docosahexaenoic acid) play an important role in maintaining balance in the body (The Nutrition Source n.d.). The most compelling evidence of omega-3 fats' benefits relates to heart disease (The Nutrition Source n.d.). These fats help maintain a steady heartbeat, reducing the risk of dangerous or potentially fatal irregular rhythms (The Nutrition Source n.d.). Such arrhythmias are responsible for the majority of the 500,000+ cardiac-related deaths in the United States each year (The Nutrition Source n.d.). Additionally, omega-3s lower blood pressure and heart rate while enhancing blood vessel function (The Nutrition Source n.d.). In higher doses, they can reduce triglyceride levels and may help alleviate inflammation, a key factor in the progression of atherosclerosis (The Nutrition Source n.d.). Omega-3s also contribute to brain health, enhancing cognitive function and potentially lowering the risk of depression.

But omega-3s are just the beginning of what salmon offers. This fish is packed with essential nutrients beyond its healthy fats. Selenium, a mineral found in salmon, is vital for thyroid health and acts as an antioxidant, further protecting cells from damage. Salmon is also rich in B vitamins, which are vital for energy production, DNA repair, and reducing inflammation. These vitamins support a range of bodily functions, ensuring that you have the energy and resilience to tackle daily challenges. The combination of these nutrients makes salmon a high value nutritional food.

Studies have highlighted the anti-inflammatory effects of salmon. Research shows that regular consumption of salmon can lower inflammatory markers and improve joint health, particularly in individuals with arthritis (The Nutrition Source n.d.). The omega-3s in salmon are shown to ease joint stiffness and reduce tenderness, providing relief for those struggling with arthritic pain (The Nutrition Source n.d.)

Selecting and preparing salmon wisely is necessary for maximizing its health benefits. When shopping, choose wild-caught salmon over farmed varieties. Wild-caught salmon generally contains higher levels of omega-3s and fewer contaminants, such as PCBs and mercury, which are sometimes found in farmed fish. This choice ensures you are getting the best nutritional value while minimizing potential health risks. When it comes to preparation, consider baking or grilling salmon to preserve its nutrients and keep it deliciously moist. These methods enhance the natural flavors of the fish without adding unnecessary calories. Season your salmon with herbs and lemon juice for a simple but flavorful dish that supports your health goals.

Quinoa: The Ancient Grain for Modern Health

Unlike most grains, quinoa is a complete protein, meaning it contains all nine essential amino acids that our bodies cannot produce on their own (Kubala and Gunnars 2024). This makes it particularly valuable for vegetarians and vegans who might struggle to get these amino acids from a plant-based diet. Two key amino acids found in quinoa are lysine and methionine. Lysine is important for tissue growth and repair, while methionine plays a central role in metabolism and detoxification. This complete amino acid profile makes quinoa an effective nutritional choice.

Beyond its protein content, quinoa contains anti-inflammatory properties that can help keep your body in balance. It is high in fiber, which enhances digestion and plays a role in reducing inflammation (Kubala and Gunnars 2024). Fiber helps feed the good bacteria in your gut, which in turn can reduce inflammation throughout the body. Quinoa is also a good source of magnesium, a mineral known to combat inflammation and support muscle and nerve function (Kubala and Gunnars 2024). These nutrients work together to provide a powerful anti-inflammatory effect, helping to soothe chronic inflammation and promote better health.

Additionally, quinoa's gentle impact on blood sugar levels makes it a smart choice for those managing diabetes or insulin resistance. Its fiber content slows down digestion, leading to a more gradual release of glucose into the bloodstream. This helps keep blood sugar levels stable, reducing the risk of spikes and crashes that can lead to inflammation (Kubala and Gunnars 2024).

One of quinoa's biggest advantages is its versatility in the kitchen. It can easily replace rice or pasta in many dishes, providing a nutritious alternative that does not skimp on flavor. You might also try using quinoa as a base for salads and hot or cold bowls, mixing it with fresh vegetables, herbs, and a dressing of your choice for a satisfying meal. Its mild, nutty flavor pairs well with a variety of ingredients, making it a great addition to any meal. You can also use quinoa to make a hearty breakfast porridge, adding fruits, nuts, and a drizzle of honey for sweetness. By experimenting with quinoa in different dishes, you can keep your meals interesting and nutrient-rich.

Leafy Greens: Nutrient-Dense and Delicious

Leafy greens are nature's multivitamin. Spinach, kale, and their leafy relatives, Swiss chard and collard greens, are loaded with vitamins, minerals, and phytochemicals that are important for reducing inflammation. Vitamin A, abundant in leafy greens, is vital for vision, immune function, and skin health (Healthdirect n.d.). It acts as an antioxidant, protecting your cells from damage. Folate, another key nutrient, supports DNA synthesis and repair, which is required for cell growth and function (U.S. Centers for Disease Control and Prevention n.d.). This vitamin is particularly important for women who are pregnant or planning to become pregnant, as it helps prevent neural tube defects in developing fetuses (U.S. Centers for Disease Control and Prevention n.d.). Leafy greens are also packed with calcium, which is crucial for strong bones and teeth, as well as iron. It is also necessary for transporting oxygen throughout the body. Together, these nutrients make leafy greens a necessary addition to your diet.

The anti-inflammatory effects of leafy greens are well-documented, thanks to their rich nutrient profile. Chlorophyll, the pigment responsible for its vibrant green color, has been shown to have anti-inflammatory, anti-cancer, and anti-obesity properties (Ebrahimi et al. 2023). Chlorophyll neutralizes toxins in the body, reducing inflammation and supporting overall health. The fiber content in leafy greens also has a role in inflammation reduction. It promotes healthy digestion and supports the growth of beneficial gut bacteria, both of which can help reduce inflammation in the body.

Exploring the variety and preparation of leafy greens can open up a world of culinary possibilities. While spinach and kale are popular choices, do not forget about other greens like Arugula, Swiss chard, and collard greens. Each offers a unique flavor and texture, allowing you to mix things up in the kitchen. Enjoy them raw in salads or smoothies for a fresh and unique taste. Pairing greens with fruits like apples or berries in a salad can create a delightful contrast of flavors. If you prefer a warmer dish, try lightly sautéing them with garlic and olive oil. This simple preparation method enhances their flavor while preserving their nutrients. You can also add any of these greens to soups and stews, where they absorb the flavors of the broth and other ingredients. By experimenting with different types and preparations, you can discover new and exciting ways to enjoy leafy greens every day.

More specifically, you might start by using leafy greens as a base for grain bowls. Combine a generous handful of greens with quinoa, roasted vegetables, and your choice of protein for a balanced and satisfying meal. You can also blend greens into your morning smoothie for an added nutrient boost. Just a handful of spinach or kale can seamlessly blend into a fruit smoothie, providing all the benefits without altering the taste. Another easy way to add greens to your meals is by tossing them into pasta dishes or casseroles. As the greens wilt, they blend into the dish, adding nutrients without overwhelming the palate.

Turmeric: Golden Spice for Inflammation

Curcumin, the vibrant yellow compound in turmeric, is where this spice gets its mighty anti-inflammatory reputation. It works by modulating the activity of molecules that play a key role in inflammation, such as cytokines and enzymes (Sharifi-Rad et al. 2020). This modulation means that curcumin can effectively reduce inflammation by interrupting the signals that tell your body to mount an inflammatory response (Sharifi-Rad et al. 2020). It is a natural way to dial down the body's overreaction, which is often at the heart of chronic inflammatory conditions.

For centuries, turmeric has been a staple in Ayurvedic medicine, where it is used to treat a variety of ailments, from digestive issues to joint pain (Sharifi-Rad et al. 2020). In these traditional practices, turmeric is a healing agent, valued for its ability to balance the body and mind (Sharifi-Rad et al. 2020). Today, turmeric has found its way into modern health diets around the world, celebrated for its potential to improve health and prevent disease. Its uses are varied and include everything from spice in cooking to a supplement in capsule form. This ancient spice has been thrust into the limelight as a modern-day superfood and for a good reason.

Scientific research has explored turmeric's benefits, particularly its effect on inflammation. Studies have shown that curcumin can reduce symptoms of inflammatory diseases, such as arthritis (Peng et al. 2021). The impact on arthritis is quite remarkable, with some studies suggesting that curcumin's anti-inflammatory effects are comparable to those of some pharmaceutical anti-inflammatory drugs (Peng et al. 2021). This research highlights the potential for turmeric to be a natural alternative or complement to traditional treatments.

Incorporating turmeric into your diet can be both delicious and health-promoting. One popular way is through golden milk, a warm, comforting beverage made with milk (or a dairy-free alternative), turmeric, and spices like cinnamon and ginger. It is not only soothing but also a great way to start or end your day with a health boost. Turmeric teas are another option, as they offer a gentle, flavorful way to enjoy this spice. In the kitchen, turmeric is incredibly versatile. Add it to curries to enhance their color and flavor, or sprinkle it into rice dishes for an aromatic twist. Its warm, earthy taste complements a wide range of foods, making it an easy addition to many meals.

Experimenting with turmeric in your cooking can open up new culinary adventures. Try making a turmeric-spiced soup or use it as a rub for grilled meats. You can even add a pinch to your scrambled eggs for a morning pick-me-up. The possibilities are endless, and each dish you create will support your health. By incorporating turmeric into your diet, you are tapping into an ancient tradition with modern benefits, helping to keep inflammation at bay while enjoying the flavors of this golden spice.

Nuts and Seeds: Crunchy Allies Against Inflammation

Nuts and seeds, though small, can significantly impact your health, particularly when it comes to inflammation. These tiny foods contain healthy fats, fiber, and protein, making them an integral part of an anti-inflammatory diet. Walnuts, for example, are rich in omega-3 fatty acids, which are known for their ability to reduce inflammation. These fats are critical for brain health and can help manage heart disease risk factors. Almonds, on the other hand, are an excellent source of Vitamin E, an antioxidant that protects cells from oxidative stress and promotes skin health. This vitamin also plays a role in reducing inflammation, making almonds a great snack choice. Besides these, nuts and seeds provide a variety of other nutrients, including magnesium and zinc, which further support overall health.

The anti-inflammatory properties of nuts and seeds are largely due to the presence of specific compounds that actively combat inflammation. Take flax seeds, for instance, which are high in alpha-linolenic acid (ALA), a type of omega-3 fatty acid (Ajmera 2024). ALA reduces inflammatory markers and improves heart health (Ajmera 2024). This makes flax seeds a valuable addition to your diet. Moreover, the fiber content in nuts and seeds plays a central role in maintaining gut health, which indirectly reduces inflammation. By supporting a healthy gut microbiome, fiber helps to lower systemic inflammation, benefiting your entire body. This combination of healthy fats, fiber, and anti-inflammatory compounds makes nuts and seeds a formidable ally in your fight against inflammation. With 3 to 7 grams of protein per ounce, nuts and seeds help fuel muscle maintenance and repair while at the same time helping to protect your brain.

Incorporating nuts and seeds into your daily routine is both simple and versatile. They can easily be added to a variety of meals and snacks. Try sprinkling a handful of chopped nuts over your salads or yogurt for a satisfying crunch and nutritional boost. You can also blend nut butters into smoothies for a creamy texture and added protein. These nut butters serve as a great base for smoothies, providing healthy fats that keep you full and energized. If you are looking for a savory option, consider using seeds like chia or pumpkin seeds in your soups or stews. Their subtle flavor and nutrient content enhance any dish, making them a valuable addition to your culinary repertoire.

While nuts and seeds offer numerous health benefits, it is important to be mindful of portion sizes to avoid consuming too many calories. A recommended serving size is about a small handful, roughly 1 ounce (1/4 cup or 28 grams). This portion provides the necessary nutrients without overloading on calories. It is also wise to rotate different types of nuts and seeds in your diet for a diverse intake of nutrients. By varying your choices, you can enjoy the benefits each type offers, from the heart-healthy fats in walnuts to the vitamin E in almonds. This variety keeps your meals interesting while also maximizing the health benefits you receive from these foods.

If you prefer roasted nuts to raw, dry-roast (no oil) @ 300 degrees F for about 10 to 25 minutes, depending on the type of nut. In the next chapter, we will explore the secrets to longevity in Mediterranean diets.

Chapter 4

The Mediterranean Diet—Secrets to Longevity

Picture a sun-drenched table set with colorful dishes, the air filled with laughter, and the aroma of fresh herbs. This scene embodies the Mediterranean lifestyle, where meals are celebrations of life. This approach to living goes beyond what is on your plate, encompassing a holistic view that prioritizes balance, community, and well-being. It is not just about the diet, but rather, it is about how life is lived.

The Mediterranean Way

The Mediterranean lifestyle encourages social eating, where meals are shared experiences, enhancing connections and community bonds. This tradition of communal meals promotes emotional well-being and encourages mindful eating, where every bite is savored and appreciated. Physical activity is another foundation of the Mediterranean lifestyle. It is focused on integrating movement into daily life. Think leisurely walks through picturesque landscapes or cycling to the local market. These activities are woven into the fabric of everyday routines, promoting health without the need for structured exercise regimens. The idea is to keep active in a way that is enjoyable and sustainable, encouraging a lifelong commitment to physical wellness. This natural incorporation of movement supports cardiovascular health and helps maintain a healthy weight, both vital components for longevity (Dominguez et al. 2024).

Daily habits in the Mediterranean lifestyle emphasize moderation, balance, and self-control in various aspects of life. Instead of rigid diets or extreme restrictions, there is an appreciation for enjoying a diverse range of foods in appropriate portions. This balanced approach allows for occasional indulgence without guilt, creating a positive relationship with food. Relaxation and stress reduction are also of significant importance. Taking time to unwind, whether through afternoon siestas or leisurely conversations with friends, helps manage stress levels and promotes mental clarity. These practices contribute to a reduced risk of chronic stress-related conditions (Dominguez et al. 2024).

Family and community play central roles in this lifestyle, as they offer emotional support and enhance mental health. Regular family gatherings and shared meals strengthen bonds and create a sense of belonging. These interactions are opportunities to connect, share stories, and express gratitude. This sense of community is linked to improved mental health outcomes, providing a buffer against loneliness and depression (Dominguez et al. 2024). By prioritizing these connections, the Mediterranean lifestyle promotes resilience and emotional well-being.

Incorporating Mediterranean practices into modern life is more feasible than it might seem. You can begin by embracing mindful eating, where you focus on the taste, texture, and enjoyment of each meal. This practice can deepen your appreciation for food and enhance your dining experience. Additionally, you might consider adopting leisurely walks as part of your routine. Whether it is a stroll through your neighborhood or a hike in nature, these walks offer physical and mental health benefits. They provide an opportunity to disconnect from digital distractions and reconnect with the natural world.

Interactive Element: Mindful Eating Exercise

As you prepare your next meal, take a moment to engage all your senses. Notice the colors, aromas, and textures of the ingredients. As you eat, chew slowly and savor each bite, paying attention to the flavors and how they make you feel. This exercise encourages a deeper connection with your food and can help enhance your enjoyment and satisfaction.

Olive Oil: Liquid Gold for Heart and Joint Health

Olive oil, often referred to as liquid gold, is a pillar of the Mediterranean diet. It is a source of healthy fats that set this diet apart. Rich in monounsaturated fatty acids, particularly oleic acid, olive oil plays a key role in maintaining heart health. This balance is important for keeping your arteries clear and your heart pumping smoothly. But olive oil doesn't stop there. It is packed with powerful antioxidants like vitamin E and polyphenols, which fight oxidative stress and inflammation in the body (Philpott 2023).

The health benefits of olive oil are well-documented, particularly its impact on cardiovascular and joint health. Studies have shown that regular consumption of olive oil is linked to a reduction in LDL cholesterol levels. This means a lower risk of heart disease, making it a smart choice for those looking to protect their heart. Olive oil's anti-inflammatory properties are another feather in its cap. Due to compounds like oleocanthal, which acts similarly to ibuprofen, olive oil can help reduce inflammation and pain. Recent studies have indicated that it could play a role in mitigating diseases such as joint degeneration, neurodegenerative disorders, and specific types of cancer (Philpott 2023).

When it comes to selecting olive oil, not all bottles are created equal. Extra virgin olive oil (EVOO) is the crème de la crème, known for its superior flavor and higher polyphenol content compared to refined versions (Philpott 2023). The process of making EVOO involves cold pressing olives, which preserves more of the natural compounds that give olive oil its health benefits. When shopping, look for labels that specify "extra virgin", "cold pressed" and organic." Also, check for harvest dates to ensure freshness. Proper storage is key to maintaining its quality. Keep your olive oil in a cool, dark place, away from heat and light, which can cause it to degrade. Using a dark glass bottle can help protect it from sunlight, keeping its flavors and nutrients intact.

Olive oil's versatility in the kitchen is unmatched. Beyond the classic salad dressing, consider drizzling it over grilled vegetables to enhance their natural flavors. The oil's fruity, peppery notes add depth to all dishes. Baking with olive oil instead of butter is another way to incorporate its benefits into your meals. It provides a moist texture to baked goods and a subtle flavor that compliments both sweet and savory dishes. Try using it in cakes, muffins, or bread for a healthier twist on traditional recipes. Turn a regular cake recipe into an olive oil cake by substituting the butter or shortening with olive oil, using about ¾ cup EVOO for every cup of butter/shortening.

Another creative use of olive oil is in marinades for meats or tofu, where it helps tenderize and infuse flavors. Its high smoke point makes it suitable for sautéing and light frying, offering a healthier alternative to other cooking oils. Even a simple dip of olive oil with balsamic vinegar or herbs and spices can elevate a loaf of crusty bread, turning a basic snack into a gourmet starter. These culinary uses highlight olive oil's adaptability and guarantee that you are getting its health benefits with every meal.

Fresh Produce: Fruits and Vegetables at the Core

The Mediterranean diet, with an abundance of fresh produce at its core, embraces the concept that fruits and vegetables are central to each meal. Seasonal and locally sourced produce is important to this diet, making sure that what you eat is fresh, flavorful, and packed with nutrients. By choosing locally grown seasonal produce, you get the best flavors and the most nutrients, as fruits and vegetables are harvested at their peak. This supports your health and contributes to sustainable agriculture by reducing the carbon footprint of transporting foods over long distances.

The nutritional benefits of fresh produce are significant. Citrus fruits, for example, contain vitamin C, a powerful antioxidant that supports your immune system and helps keep your skin glowing (Jennings 2023). This vitamin also supports collagen production, which is critical for healthy skin and joints. Tomatoes, a staple in Mediterranean cuisine, contain lycopene, which is a potent antioxidant that protects cells from damage caused by free radicals (Bjarnadottir 2023). They are also rich in potassium, a mineral that helps regulate blood pressure and supports heart health (Bjarnadottir 2023). Potassium also plays a role in muscle function and nerve signaling, making it a vital nutrient for overall well-being (Bjarnadottir 2023). The fiber found in many fruits and vegetables is another key component, enhancing digestion and reducing the risk of chronic diseases. By integrating a wide variety of fruits and vegetables into your diet, you are nourishing your body with essential nutrients that support every aspect of your health.

When looking to maximize your fresh produce intake, you might start by preparing colorful salads that showcase a variety of textures and flavors. Combine leafy greens with vegetables like bell peppers, cucumbers, and radishes. Add fruits like berries or slices of citrus for a hint of sweetness and a burst of vitamin C. Another strategy is to make vegetable-heavy stews, where the vegetables take center stage. Use a variety of veggies, such as zucchini, eggplant, and tomatoes, simmered with herbs and spices for a warming, hearty meal.

Eating seasonally is a concept that is also gaining traction contemporarily. Seasonal produce is often more affordable, more flavorful, and more nutritious. When fruits and vegetables are in season, they are at their natural best, offering superior taste and texture. Eating seasonally also encourages variety in your diet, as different fruits and vegetables come into season at different times of the year. In the spring, you might enjoy tender asparagus and sweet strawberries, while in the fall, you can savor the rich flavors of squash and apples. This variety guarantees that your diet is diverse and balanced, providing a wide range of nutrients that support your health. Seasonal eating also connects you to the natural rhythms of the earth, establishing a deeper appreciation for the food you eat and where it comes from.

To incorporate more seasonal produce into your life, consider visiting local farmers' markets, where you can find fresh, locally grown fruits and vegetables. These markets offer a chance to connect with local farmers and learn more about the produce you are buying. You will often find unique varieties that are not available in supermarkets, adding diversity and excitement to your meals. By prioritizing seasonal produce, you are enhancing your meals while also supporting local agriculture and promoting sustainability. This simple shift in perspective can make a big difference in both your health and the health of the planet.

Whole Grains: Staple Foods for Sustained Energy

Whole grains are the backbone of a balanced diet. Each grain comprises three parts: bran, germ, and endosperm. The bran is where most of the fiber is, providing roughage that aids digestion. The germ houses essential fats, vitamins, and antioxidants, while the endosperm contains carbohydrates and protein for energy. Together, these components make whole grains a nutritional powerhouse, offering a steady release of energy, unlike highly processed refined grains that are stripped of these nutrients. This means whole grains keep you fuller for longer and provide a sustained energy release, ideal for tackling your day without the afternoon slump (Oldways Whole Grains Council n.d.).

The health benefits of whole grains are significant. Because of their high fiber content, they support digestion by promoting regular bowel movements and preventing constipation. This fiber sweeps through your digestive tract and keeps everything moving smoothly. Fiber is also known to lower cholesterol levels, reducing the risk of heart disease. The slow-release carbohydrates in whole grains help maintain stable blood sugar levels, providing a steady supply of energy without spikes and crashes. This is particularly beneficial for those looking to manage their weight or those with diabetes. Additionally, without the bran and germ, about 25% of a grain's protein is lost and is greatly reduced in at least seventeen key nutrients (Oldways Whole Grains Council n.d.). Overall, whole grains are healthier, providing more protein, more fiber, and many important vitamins and minerals (Oldways Whole Grains Council n.d.)

In the Mediterranean diet, common whole grains include barley, farro, and bulgur. Barley is versatile and can be used in soups, salads, and stews. It has a chewy texture and nutty flavor, making it a hearty addition to any meal. Farro, an ancient grain, is rich in nutrients and offers a chewiness that pairs well with roasted vegetables or meats. It is often used in salads or as a base for grain bowls. Bulgur, a quick-cooking whole grain, is a useful ingredient in dishes like tabbouleh. It has a light, nutty flavor and a fluffy texture, perfect for absorbing the flavors of herbs and spices. These grains add texture and flavor to meals while also providing a wealth of nutrients that support overall health.

Incorporating whole grains into your diet does not have to be complicated. Start by replacing refined grains with whole grains in your meals. Swap white rice for brown rice or quinoa and choose whole-grain bread instead of white bread. These small changes can make a big difference in your nutrient intake. Experiment with different cooking methods to bring out the best in each grain. For instance, try simmering barley in broth for a flavorful side dish or roasting farro with vegetables for a warm salad. Bulgur is a whole wheat product, usually durum wheat, that is made from wheat kernels that have been cleaned, boiled, dried, and cracked into small pieces. Bulgur can be soaked in hot water for a quick addition to salads or used as a base for a nutritious bowl. Just note that durum wheat is a type of wheat that is high in both protein and gluten, so it is usually used to make bread and pasta.

Visual Element: Whole Grain Cooking Chart

This chart outlines the cooking times and methods for different whole grains. This is a handy reference that will help you prepare these grains effectively every time.

Whole Grain Cooking Chart

Grain	Water Ratio	Cooking Time	Yield	Notes
White Rice	1:2	15-20 min	3 cups	Rinse before cooking
Brown Rice	1:2.5	40-45 min	3 cups	Nutty flavor, more nutrients
Quinoa	1:2	15-20 min	3 cups	Rinse well to remove saponins
Oats (rolled)	1:2	5-10 min	2 cups	Quick-cooking breakfast option
Steel-cut Oats	1:3	20-30 min	3 cups	Chewy texture, nutty flavor
Barley (pearled)	1:3	40-50 min	3.5 cups	Great in soups and stews
Bulgur	1:2	10-15 min	2.5 cups	Often used in tabbouleh
Millet	1:2.5	25-30 min	3.5 cups	Light, fluffy texture
Farro	1:3	30-40 min	3 cups	Chewy texture, nutty flavor
Couscous	1:1.5	5-10 min	2.5 cups	Not a true grain, but pasta
Wild Rice	1:3	45-55 min	3.5 cups	Actually an aquatic grass seed
Amaranth	1:2.5	20-25 min	2.5 cups	Tiny grains, slightly sweet
Buckwheat	1:2	15-20 min	2.5 cups	Great for breakfast porridge

Cooking Tips:

- Ratios are 1 cup of grain to water by volume
- Bring water to boil, add grain, reduce to simmer, cover
- Let grains rest 5-10 minutes after cooking
- Salt to taste (typically ¼ tsp per cup of dry grain)

Legumes and Beans: Plant-Based Protein Powerhouses

When you think of a satisfying and nutritious meal, legumes and beans should come to mind. They are central to plant-based diets, offering a robust source of protein. Their fiber content also enhances digestion, keeps you feeling full longer, and helps maintain steady blood sugar levels. This combination of protein and fiber makes legumes and beans a staple in many cultures, providing essential nutrients without the need for animal products.

The health benefits of legumes and beans are as diverse as their varieties. One of their standout qualities is their ability to support heart health. By incorporating them into your diet, you can help lower cholesterol levels due to their soluble fiber content. This type of fiber binds to cholesterol in the digestive system, helping to remove it from the body and reduce the risk of heart disease. Additionally, legumes and beans are rich in antioxidants, which combat oxidative stress and inflammation in the body. These antioxidants protect your cells from damage and reduce the risk of chronic diseases (American Heart Association 2025).

In Mediterranean cuisine, legumes and beans are celebrated for their flavor. Chickpeas, for example, are a popular choice, often added to salads or used in dishes like soups and stews or blended to make hummus even roasted for a crunchy chickpea snack. Lentils, another favorite, come in various colors and can be used in soups, stews, or salads. Their quick cooking time and ability to absorb flavors make them a convenient and delicious addition to any meal. Fava beans, with their rich, buttery texture, are often used in traditional Mediterranean dishes, offering a unique flavor profile that pairs well with herbs and spices. These legumes are nutritious and provide a base for many meals, making them a valuable ingredient in any kitchen.

Incorporating legumes and beans into your meals can be a fun and creative process. Consider making a batch of homemade hummus by blending chickpeas with tahini, lemon juice, and roasted garlic. Make a sweet red pepper hummus by adding a roasted red bell pepper, a little olive oil and a little sriracha in the blender with the chickpeas. This creamy dip is perfect for spreading on sandwiches or serving with fresh vegetables. To make a tasty appetizer, grill some french bread slices, spread on any flavor of hummus and top with roasted veggies, feta cheese or fresh herbs.

If you are in the mood for something warm and comforting, try adding lentils to your favorite soup or stew. They provide a satisfying texture and earthy flavor that goes well with a variety of ingredients. For a fresh and vibrant dish, toss together a bean salad with your choice of legumes, diced vegetables, and a light vinaigrette. This salad is not only healthy but also refreshing, making it an ideal side dish or light lunch.

Beans and legumes are also perfect for hearty winter stews. The beans soak up all the flavors in the broth while adding a satisfying bite. You can even incorporate them into your breakfast routine. Consider making a savory breakfast bowl with black beans, avocado, some salsa and a poached egg for a protein-packed start to your day. For a twist on traditional dishes, try using white beans as a base for a creamy sauce, adding them to pasta or casseroles. Their mild flavor allows them to blend seamlessly into a variety of recipes, offering a nutritious boost without overpowering the dish.

Herbs and Spices: Flavorful Ways to Fight Inflammation

Herbs and spices elevate the flavors of your meals while also containing an array of health benefits, making them a staple in the Mediterranean diet. They have been used for centuries to enhance taste and promote wellness. They contain antioxidant properties that protect your cells from damage and reduce inflammation.

In the Mediterranean diet, specific herbs and spices are celebrated for their anti-inflammatory prowess. Basil, with its sweet and slightly peppery flavor, is more than just a garnish. It contains eugenol, a compound known for its anti-inflammatory effects. Add it to pasta, blend it with olive oil, pine nuts, and parmesan to make a zesty pesto sauce, or wrap it around a cherry tomato and ball of mozzarella for a Caprese appetizer. My favorite way to use extra pesto sauce is to spread on a crunchy baguette roll with fresh tuna salad. Oregano, another kitchen favorite, is rich in antioxidants and offers antimicrobial benefits, making it a powerful herb that supports immune health. Oregano also belongs in every tomato sauce, from marinara to puttanesca. Rosemary, with its earthy aroma, is packed with rosmarinic acid, which reduces inflammation. Sprinkle rosemary copiously on salmon filets or roasted red potatoes for an elevated flavor profile (Dryfo n.d.).

The health benefits of incorporating these herbs and spices into your diet are significant. Their anti-inflammatory compounds can help reduce swelling and pain, especially in chronic inflammatory diseases. By including them in your meals, you are taking a natural and delicious approach to managing inflammation and supporting your health. These herbs and spices also add depth and complexity to dishes, making healthy eating an enjoyable and flavorful experience. Also, they can help reduce the need for added salt and sugar, contributing to a more balanced and nutritious diet.

To make the most of these herbs and spices, consider how you might incorporate them into your cooking. Fresh herbs often have more flavor compared to their dried counterparts, so if you have the option, try using fresh basil, oregano, or rosemary in your dishes as a garnish or topping. They can be easily snipped from a garden or bought fresh from the market. However, dried herbs have their place, too, offering convenience and a more concentrated flavor, perfect for slow-cooked dishes. Another way to enjoy the benefits of herbs is by infusing oils. You might utilize a bottle of olive oil infused with rosemary or garlic, which is useful for drizzling over roasted vegetables or as a dipping sauce for bread. Add some garlic for extra anti-inflammatory impact. These infused oils add flavor and carry the health benefits of the herbs.

Experimenting with these ingredients can open up a world of culinary possibilities. Instead of relying on heavy sauces or salt, try seasoning your dishes with a blend of spices. For instance, delicate saffron threads create a luxurious risotto or paella, where its subtle flavor shines. Incorporating herbs and spices into your daily meals can be an effective way to enhance your diet and protect your health. The next chapter explores the importance of personalized anti-inflammatory diet plans, along with some examples and ideas for you to try out.

Chapter 5

Personalized Anti-Inflammatory Diet Plans

It is you who holds the power to choose whether to take the path leading to improved health or the other path of your same old routine. Years of eating a standard American diet (SAD) might have you questioning whether it is time to take charge of your health and make improvements. This is where crafting a personalized anti-inflammatory meal plan is useful. It focuses on creating a meal plan that is tailored to your own tastes, needs, and goals. Whether you are aiming to manage your weight, boost your energy, or simply feel better on a day-to-day basis, understanding your dietary goals is the first step.

Creating Your Own Meal Plan

First, you need to identify what you want to achieve with your diet. Perhaps weight management is at the top of your list. If so, consider how your current eating habits align with this goal. Are you consuming more calories than your body needs, or are you not getting enough nutrients to support a healthy metabolism? On the other hand, if improving energy levels is your primary focus, examine how your meals impact your mood and stamina. Are you feeling sluggish after eating, or do certain foods leave you feeling energized? Taking time to reflect on these questions will help you set clear, realistic objectives that guide your meal planning.

Once you have set your goals, it is time to design a meal plan that will help you achieve these goals. Think of it as assembling a puzzle, where each piece represents an element of your diet. Balancing macronutrients—proteins, fats, and carbohydrates—is key to creating satisfying, nourishing meals. Aim to include a source of each macronutrient in every meal, adjusting portions to align with your goals. Variety is another important factor, working to prevent monotony and ensure the utility of a wide range of nutrients. Incorporate different fruits, vegetables, grains, and proteins throughout the week, keeping your meals new and exciting.

Meal plans are not set in stone; rather, they require flexibility and adjustment as you progress. Pay attention to how your body responds to changes in your diet. Keeping a food journal is important in tracking progress and making necessary adjustments. Note what you eat, how you feel, and any changes in your health. From there, tweak your meal plan as needed. Perhaps you need more protein to stay full longer, or maybe reducing portion sizes of certain foods can help with weight management. These observations will guide you in refining your plan.

To help you get started, here is a sample one-week meal plan template with a focus on anti-inflammatory foods:

When creating a personalized meal plan, incorporate the following into your breakfast, lunch, and dinner:

- Choose a high protein, low gluten grain as the base (oats, quinoa, brown rice, or sprouted-grain toast like Ezekiel bread).
- Add some superfood greens, (sauteed spinach, arugula, kale, chard).
- Add protein (egg, grilled chicken or fish).
- Add healthy fat (olive oil, avocado).
- Add some healthy nuts and/or seeds (walnuts, almonds, pecans, pine nuts).

Seasonal Meal Plan Variation

Consider adapting your meal plan to the seasons to take advantage of fresh, local produce. In spring, incorporate asparagus and peas; in summer, enjoy tomatoes and zucchini; in fall, savor squash and apples; and in winter, turn to root vegetables and citrus fruits. This approach supports local agriculture while also keeping your diet diverse and nutrient-rich.

Creating a meal plan is an evolving process, one that changes as you learn more about your body's needs and preferences. It is about finding what works for you, making adjustments along the way, and enjoying the journey to better health.

Personally I was amazed when I started feeling less hungry all the time and my energy levels and sleep patterns improved after just a few weeks of following a diet based on superfoods. I could see a commercial about juicy fried chicken or cheeseburgers and fries without feeling like I needed to have that right now. Just seeing food would make me think I was hungry and trigger a snack attack, but now it has no impact and I just carry protein bars or homemade granola with me when I think I might be too busy to eat.

Quick and Easy Meal Prep: Solutions for Busy Lives

In the hustle and bustle of daily life, staying on track with your dietary goals can feel overwhelming. Between work, family, and social commitments, cooking healthy meals can easily slip to the bottom of the priority list. This is where meal prepping becomes a game-changer. By planning and preparing meals in advance, you will save valuable time during the week and reduce stress so that you can stick to your anti-inflammatory diet. Imagine coming home after a long day to a fridge stocked with ready-to-eat meals that align with your health goals. This is both a convenient and a practical approach to maintaining a healthy lifestyle amid the chaos.

The key to successful meal prep lies in organization and efficiency. Start by setting aside a specific day for planning and prepping your meals. Many people find Sundays ideal for this task, giving them a head start on a busy week ahead. Begin with batch cooking, where you make large quantities of food that can be used in multiple meals. Think hearty vegetable stews or roasted chicken that can be shredded and added to salads or wraps. As you cook, portion out meals into individual containers, making them easy to grab and go. Investing in a set of quality meal prep containers can make a world of difference. Look for ones that are microwave-safe and have secure lids to keep your food fresh.

Freezing meals is another useful strategy for those days when you simply do not have time to cook. Soups, casseroles, and even cooked grains can be frozen and reheated easily. When freezing, be sure to allow food to cool completely before sealing it in airtight containers or freezer bags. This prevents ice crystals from forming and makes sure that your meals taste just as good when reheated. Label each container with the contents and date so you always know what is available. Having a freezer stocked with nutritious meals means you are never more than a few minutes away from a healthy dinner.

For those of us with jam-packed schedules, quick recipes are life-savers. One-pan meals, for instance, are perfect for saving time and reducing cleanup. Consider a sheet-pan dinner with salmon, sweet potatoes, and broccoli, all seasoned with olive oil and herbs. Drizzle the sweet potatoes with olive oil and put them in the oven first. Add the salmon and salmon filets after about 45 minutes and it's all done within 15 minutes more. Everything cooks together, blending flavors beautifully. Overnight oats are another simple option for breakfast. Mix oats with almond milk, chia seeds, and your favorite fruits, and let them soak in the fridge overnight. These oats save time in the morning and provide a nutritious start to your day.

Equipping your kitchen with the right tools can further streamline the meal prep process. Slow cookers and pressure cookers are useful for making large batches of food with minimal effort. They allow you to set it and forget it, perfect for busy days. A pressure cooker can turn a tough cut of meat into a tender dish in under an hour, while a slow cooker can simmer a stew all day, ready for you when you return home. Meal prep containers, as mentioned earlier, are helpful. Having a variety of sizes helps you portion meals correctly, avoiding waste and making sure that you have the right amount for each serving.

Meal prepping is both saving time and setting yourself up for success. With a little planning and preparation, you can create a routine that supports your health goals while fitting seamlessly into your lifestyle. It is a simple but effective way to take control of your diet, reduce weekday stress, and enjoy the benefits of an anti-inflammatory lifestyle.

Budget-Friendly Anti-inflammatory Ingredients

Eating healthy does not have to break the bank. When you are on a budget, it is important to make smart choices that maximize nutrition without depleting your wallet. Oatmeal is a breakfast mainstay, and you can jazz it up with nuts, seeds, a couple of chopped dates, or a tablespoon of dark chocolate chips. For lunch or dinner, start with canned beans, chickpeas, or lentils, which are pantry staples that pack a punch in terms of protein and fiber. They are incredibly versatile, fitting seamlessly into soups, salads, and stews. You can whip up a hearty lentil soup or a simple bean salad, both of which are filling and nutritious. Grains like farro, barley, brown rice, and quinoa can be bought in bulk and stored for extended periods of time. Seasonal fruits and vegetables are another great choice. Not only are they typically less expensive when in season, but they also taste better and are fresher. Think of the crispness of apples in the fall or the juiciness of tomatoes in the summer. Buying what is local and in season can save you money while providing your body with the nutrients it craves.

Shopping smart is the key to sticking to your budget. Buying in bulk is another useful strategy. Items like grains, nuts, and seeds often cost less per unit when purchased in larger quantities. Consider visiting bulk food stores where you can buy just the amount you need, reducing waste and cost. Do not overlook sales and discounts, either. Keep an eye on weekly flyers and stock up on items when they are on sale. This approach requires a bit of planning but can lead to significant savings over time. Another tip is to compare prices between brands and stores. Sometimes, opting for a store brand or visiting a different supermarket can make a big difference in your grocery bill.

When it comes to budget-friendly meal ideas, simplicity reigns supreme. Hearty vegetable soups are comforting and economical.

Use vegetables that are in season or on sale, and add some quinoa, along with lentils or beans for protein. A big pot can last a few days, providing multiple meals. Rice and bean dishes are another staple, and they are filling, nutritious, and cost-effective. Add spices, herbs, and a squeeze of lime to elevate the flavors. These meals are easy on the wallet and also kind to your body, supporting an anti-inflammatory lifestyle.

Meal planning is a strong tool for managing food costs. By planning your meals in advance, you can create a focused shopping list that helps you avoid impulse buys. This practice keeps you within budget and reduces food waste. When you know exactly what you need for the week, you are less likely to let food spoil in the fridge. Consider setting aside time each week to plan your meals, taking into account what you already have on hand. This habit can lead to more mindful shopping and eating, benefiting both your health and your finances.

Weekly Budget Meal Plan Template

This simple chart lays out breakfast, lunch, dinner, and snacks for a week, complete with a shopping list. Here, visualizing your meals can make the planning process more tangible and enjoyable. This is a small step that can have a big impact on your wallet and your well-being.

Anti-Inflammatory Superfood Weekly Meal Plan

Day	Breakfast	Lunch	Dinner	Snacks
Monday	Oatmeal with blueberries, walnuts, and chia seeds	Kale salad with grilled salmon, avocado, and olive oil dressing	Quinoa bowl with roasted brussels sprouts, sweet potatoes, and turmeric-ginger tofu	Greek yogurt with raspberries and hemp seeds
Tuesday	Green tea smoothie with spinach, mango, and flax seeds	Lentil soup with carrots, garlic, and dark leafy greens	Baked trout with steamed broccoli and farro	Handful of mixed nuts (almonds, pecans) and an apple
Wednesday	Greek yogurt parfait with strawberries, pomegranate seeds, and pistachios	Quinoa salad with edamame, beets, and olive oil-lemon dressing	Grilled herring with roasted cauliflower and sweet potato	Dark chocolate (70%+) and a pear
Thursday	Chia seed pudding with blackberries and Brazil nuts	Spinach wrap with tuna, avocado, and tomatoes	Black bean bowl with brown rice, kale, and guacamole	Celery with almond butter and goji berries
Friday	Scrambled eggs with mushrooms, spinach, and turmeric	Mediterranean salad with sardines, arugula, and olive oil	Grilled mackerel with roasted brussels sprouts and amaranth	Blueberries and walnuts
Saturday	Avocado toast on whole grain bread with cherry tomatoes	Bean and vegetable soup with turmeric and ginger	Baked salmon with steamed kale and quinoa	Dark chocolate covered strawberries
Sunday	Oatmeal with grated apple, cinnamon, and pumpkin seeds	Arugula salad with grilled chicken, berries, and olive oil dressing	Stir-fried tofu with broccoli, mushrooms, garlic, and ginger over brown rice	Coconut yogurt with kiwi and flax seeds

Shopping List

Produce

- Blueberries, blackberries, strawberries, raspberries
- Avocados (3-4)
- Mango, apple, pear, kiwi, pomegranate
- Goji berries
- Kale, spinach, arugula
- Brussels sprouts, broccoli, cauliflower
- Sweet potatoes (2-3)
- Carrots, beets
- Mushrooms (1 package)
- Tomatoes, cherry tomatoes
- Garlic (1 bulb)
- Fresh ginger root
- Fresh turmeric root (or ground turmeric)
- Lemons (2-3)
- Celery

Proteins

- Salmon fillets (2 packages)
- Trout fillets (1 package)
- Herring fillets (1 package)
- Mackerel fillets (1 package)
- Sardines (1 can)
- Tuna (1 can)
- Tofu (1 block)
- Chicken breast (optional)
- Eggs (1 dozen)

Grains & Legumes

- Rolled oats
- Quinoa
- Farro
- Amaranth
- Brown rice
- Whole grain bread
- Lentils
- Black beans
- Edamame (frozen)

Dairy & Alternatives

- Greek yogurt
- Coconut yogurt

Nuts, Seeds & Oils

- Walnuts, almonds, pecans, Brazil nuts, pistachios
- Chia seeds, flax seeds, hemp seeds, pumpkin seeds
- Extra virgin olive oil

Other

- Green tea
- Dark chocolate (70%+ cacao)
- Almond butter
- Spices: cinnamon, turmeric (if not using fresh)

Customize your own meal planning template by changing out the proteins, produce, grains or legumes you prefer.

Dining Out Smart: Making Healthy Choices

Eating out does not have to mean abandoning your dietary goals. Armed with a few clever strategies, you can enjoy a meal at your favorite restaurant without compromising your health. Start by scanning the menu with a discerning eye, looking for dishes that align with an anti-inflammatory diet. Select items that highlight fresh ingredients, like salads loaded with colorful vegetables, grilled fish, or lean meats. Customize your options by removing or replacing heavy fatty cheese in favor of a little feta or parmesan. These choices are often lower in unhealthy fats and sodium, making them better for your body. Do not hesitate to ask your server for modifications. Request sauces or dressings on the side to control portion size, or swap out fries for a side of pickled or steamed vegetables. Most restaurants are happy to accommodate dietary preferences, and making these small changes can significantly reduce your intake of inflammatory ingredients.

Dining out often comes with its pitfalls, and identifying these challenges is half the battle. One common trap is the allure of high-sodium and fried foods. They may taste good, but they can leave you feeling bloated and sluggish. Instead, look for menu items that are baked, grilled, or steamed. These cooking methods typically use less oil, retaining more of the food's natural nutrients and flavors. Another challenge is portion sizes, which can be much larger than what you would typically serve at home. You might decide to share a dish with a friend or ask for a to-go box when your meal arrives. This way, you can enjoy your meal without overeating.

Certain cuisines naturally align with anti-inflammatory principles, making them excellent choices when dining out. Mediterranean and Asian cuisines, for instance, emphasize whole foods, healthy fats, and lean proteins. Mediterranean dishes often feature olive oil, fish, legumes, and plenty of vegetables, all of which support an anti-inflammatory diet (Dominguez 2024). Asian cuisine, particularly Japanese and Thai, frequently includes a variety of vegetables and tofu seasoned with herbs and spices like ginger and turmeric (Indulge n.d.). These ingredients add flavor and contribute to reducing inflammation (Indulge n.d.). When possible, choose restaurants that specialize in these cuisines to find meals that align with your dietary goals more easily. Restaurant salad dressings are loaded with sugar, salt, unhealthy oils and MSG. I ask if they have olive oil and vinegar that I can put on myself or, if not, I ask for my dressing on the side and dip my fork into the dressing before spearing the lettuce, tomatoes and veggies in the salad. This way you get the flavor without overdoing it.

Special occasions and social dining can sometimes make sticking to your diet feel tricky. However, a little planning can go a long way. If you know you will be attending a dinner party or event, eat a healthy snack or a light meal beforehand to curb your appetite and prevent overindulgence. Communicate your dietary preferences with the host if you feel comfortable, and they might surprise you by accommodating your needs. If your family reunion features BBQ ribs and brisket, french fries, mashed potatoes, mac and cheese, potato salad, coleslaw loaded with dressing containing sugar, sweet tea and apple pie, you have a challenge. Don't miss out on the family connection. Eat first then put a little of everything on your plate, taste a bite if you want, then have fun visiting. Put water or tea in your travel mug to stay hydrated. If you're thinking that menu sounds like heaven you might be right, you just have to decide if you prefer a long healthy life over heaven.

When dining out with friends or family, suggest restaurants that offer a variety of healthy options. This ensures you have choices and also introduces your loved ones to delicious, nutritious meals. Remember, nobody is perfect, and it is okay to indulge occasionally as long as you make mindful choices most of the time. Eating healthy is a long-term plan. The longer you spend eating healthy, the less you will crave the unhealthy options.

Let me tell you about Joe. A lovely man whose idea of normal eating, when I met him, was a breakfast of bacon and eggs with biscuits and gravy. Lunch was a quarter pounder with fries and a chocolate shake. Dinner was a steak, baked potato with lots of butter, and several cocktails. At 38, he was 30 pounds overweight and a workaholic who traveled a lot, spending time in airport bars and having big dinners with clients until late at night with little sleep and lots of stress. His doctor said it was a perfect recipe for a heart attack by age 50, but he did not know any other way to eat. Gradually, over time, things changed. Breakfast was oatmeal with coconut flakes, cinnamon, and walnuts. Lunch became tuna sandwiches with a side salad and iced tea. Grilled salmon filets replaced the 16-ounce steaks with a side of asparagus instead of baked potato. Red wine replaced Jack Daniels. Evening walks replaced sitting in bars with colleagues. His blood pressure came down, and he even had the energy to run a few 5K and 10K races sponsored by his company. Years later, he would muse, "You know, if you hadn't changed my diet, I probably wouldn't be here now. And what's funny is I don't even miss those old food habits. The last time I had a steak, it felt like a lead weight in my stomach for days." It didn't happen overnight, but the next 38 years were much happier than the first 38 years. You can always find foods you like that will help you live a longer, healthier, happier life. It is worth the effort.

You might think that social dining scenarios with an anti-inflammatory focus might seem daunting, but with these strategies, you can maintain your dietary goals while enjoying meals out.

Embrace the opportunity to explore new cuisines and flavors that align with your health objectives and take pride in making choices that support your well-being. Eating out should not be a source of stress; instead, it should be an enjoyable experience that complements your lifestyle.

Snacking Wisely: Anti-inflammatory Options on the Go

If you start feeling that all-too-familiar energy dip around mid-day, you are not alone. Reaching for a smart snack is the best solution, providing the boost you need to keep going without the crash that often follows sugary or processed snacks. Snacking wisely is vital for maintaining energy levels and keeping hunger at bay. A well-chosen snack can prevent those energy crashes that leave you feeling sluggish and irritable. Instead of that candy bar or bag of greasy chips, choose fruit or some crunchy veggies with hummus. It is important that you consume foods that support your health and well-being throughout the day.

When it comes to anti-inflammatory snacks, simplicity is key. A mix of nuts and seeds is an effective option. They are packed with healthy fats, protein, and fiber, which help to stabilize blood sugar levels and keep you satisfied. Homemade trail mix is a great option that you can make in large batches for a week's worth of snacks. Almonds, walnuts, and sunflower seeds are all strong choices. You can carry a small bag of this mix with you whether you are heading to work or running errands. Fresh fruit paired with nut butter is another convenient and delicious snack. Apples or bananas with a spread of almond or cashew butter offer a satisfying combination of carbs and protein, ideal for a quick energy boost. These snacks are easy to pack and require minimal preparation, making them perfect for busy days.

Portion control is an important aspect of snacking that is often overlooked. Even healthy snacks can contribute to weight gain if consumed in excessive amounts. It is easy to mindlessly munch on a large bag of nuts, so try pre-portioning your snacks to avoid overconsumption. Use small containers or resealable bags to divide larger quantities into single servings. This will help with portion control and make your snacks more portable. Being mindful of portions ensures that you enjoy the benefits of snacking without unintended consequences.

Preparing snacks in advance can streamline your routine and help you stick to your dietary goals. Homemade energy bars are useful for those who enjoy a bit of weekend kitchen prep. You can make a batch using oats, nuts, seeds, and a binding agent like honey or nut butter. Not only are these bars cost-effective, but they also allow you to control the ingredients, steering clear of added sugars and preservatives often found in store-bought versions. Store them in an airtight container, and they will be ready to grab whenever you need a pick-me-up. Pre-portioned yogurt cups are another smart option. Simply divide a large tub of Greek yogurt into smaller containers and top each with fresh fruit or a sprinkle of granola. This way, you have a ready-to-eat snack that is both nourishing and satisfying.

Snacking Checklist

Start by creating a personalized snacking checklist. List your favorite anti-inflammatory snacks and preparation steps, and keep them handy as a reminder of your healthy options. Make a week's supply at a time and portion it out in portable baggies or containers. This checklist will be a quick reference, reminding you to make smart choices even on the busiest days. Need a mid-morning snack? Try ten or twelve ounces of water and yogurt with fruit and granola. Mid-afternoon dip? Reach for ten or twelve ounces of water and a handful of trail mix. These snacks will thankfully not be followed by a sugar crash that makes you feel like you really, really need a nap (SHN Staff 2022).

I have a recipe for trail mix that you can customize to taste:

- Start with whole or chopped almonds and walnuts, my favorite nuts. However, you may prefer pecans, cashews or brazil nuts.
- Next, I add either sunflower seeds or pumpkin seeds,
- Follow that with either dried banana chips or coconut flakes.
- Choose 2 or 3 dried fruits for sweetness, like cranberries, raisins, currants, papaya, apricots, pineapple, or dates (make sure your dried fruits are sulfur-free).
- And finally, just because I love dark chocolate, I add mini dark chocolate chips for a decadent flavor boost.

Depending on how much you want to make, use ½ to 1 cup of each ingredient. Mix in a large bowl and portion out into snack baggies. A serving size is about ¼ cup, which does not sound like a lot, but it is a quick snack with a lot of concentrated superfood goodness for under 200 calories and is much better for you than a candy bar.

Adapting Recipes for Dietary Restrictions

When it comes to cooking, each of us brings our own set of needs and preferences to the table. It might be due to allergies, personal choices, or health goals. Whatever the reason, adapting recipes to fit these requirements is not only possible but can also be enjoyable. For those who are gluten-sensitive or following a gluten-free diet, simple swaps can make a significant difference. Consider using almond flour or coconut flour in place of wheat flour when baking. You can get pasta made with chickpea flour, spelt, quinoa, or even hearts of palm to replace the high-gluten wheat pasta most prevalent in the United States. These alternatives maintain the desired texture and flavor without the gluten. It is possible to be sensitive to gluten, even if you are not a full-blown Celiac, and that sensitivity is very hard to diagnose. You have to prioritize what feels right for you. Similarly, if you are avoiding dairy, as I do, there are plenty of substitutes to keep your recipes creamy and satisfying. Almond milk, for instance, is an effective substitute for dairy milk. It is versatile enough to use in everything from your morning coffee to baking. Oat milk, different types of nut milks, rice milk, and soy milk give you many alternatives to find something that works best for you. Remember, these substitutions are about enhancing your meals while accommodating your needs.

For those embracing vegan or vegetarian lifestyles, modifying recipes is all about creativity. Many traditional dishes rely heavily on animal products, but with a few tweaks, you can enjoy plant-based versions. Consider using quinoa instead of couscous. Not only is quinoa gluten-free, but it also offers a complete protein source, guaranteeing that you get all the essential amino acids. It is a fantastic base for salads or as a side dish. Instead of meat, try using chickpeas or lentils for protein. These legumes are rich in nutrients and add a hearty texture to soups, stews, and even burgers. Each recipe is ready for your personal touch so that you can satisfy your personal taste.

Maintaining nutritional balance is important when adapting recipes. It is easy to cut out ingredients, but replacing their nutritional value requires a bit of thought. When you remove dairy, you might miss out on calcium. Almond milk is a useful alternative that often comes fortified with calcium and vitamin D. Similarly, if you are cutting out meat, make sure you are getting enough iron and protein from other sources like lentils, beans, and fortified cereals. It is important to make sure that each meal remains as nourishing as it is delicious so your body gets the fuel it needs to thrive.

Here are a couple of adapted recipes to give you practical examples. A vegan chickpea salad is an adjustable dish that is easy to prepare. Mix canned chickpeas with diced cucumbers, cherry tomatoes, red onion, and a handful of fresh parsley. Dress it with olive oil, lemon juice, salt, and pepper for a refreshing and protein-rich meal. Throw in some quinoa and fresh, or sauteed, super greens, and you have a supercharged, delicious, filling lunch or dinner. Another example is gluten-free pasta primavera. Use gluten-free pasta made from spelt or chickpeas, toss it with sautéed bell peppers, spinach, zucchini, and asparagus, and finish with a sprinkle of parmesan cheese or nutritional yeast for a dairy-free option. These recipes show that with a little creativity, you can enjoy meals that cater to your dietary needs without sacrificing taste or nutrition.

It is important to remember that food is meant to be enjoyed. By learning to adapt recipes, you are accommodating your own needs as well as expanding your culinary horizons. This flexibility allows you to savor a wide variety of flavors and cuisines while supporting your health goals. Whether you are cooking for yourself, your family, or friends, these adaptations guarantee that everyone can enjoy a delicious, nourishing meal together. This approach brings a sense of community and inclusivity to the table, enriching the dining experience for all involved. The next chapter discusses an array of lifestyle modifications that reduce inflammation and enhance overall health.

Chapter 6

Lifestyle Modifications for Comprehensive Health

The simple act of movement is more powerful than you might think. Exercise is an important component of maintaining a healthy and balanced life. **Beyond the well-known benefits of exercise, such as improving cardiovascular health and building muscle, regular physical activity plays a significant role in reducing inflammation.** Exercise acts as a natural anti-inflammatory agent, helping to reduce markers like C-reactive protein (CRP), which is often linked to inflammation (Kasapis and Thompson 2005). When you exercise, your circulation improves, and your lymphatic system functions better, allowing your immune cells to move efficiently through your body, enhancing their function and supporting your overall health (Kasapis and Thompson 2005).

The Importance of Exercise

A well-rounded exercise routine combines different types of activities to maximize benefits. **Aerobic exercises**, like walking, swimming, or cycling, are effective for reducing inflammation and boosting heart health. These activities get your blood pumping, which helps to lower inflammatory markers and improve circulation. **Strength training**, which includes exercises like weightlifting or resistance band workouts, plays an important role in maintaining muscle mass and bone density as we age. Additionally, **flexibility exercises**, such as yoga or Pilates, improve balance and range of motion while helping to reduce stress—another contributor to inflammation. By incorporating a combination of these exercises, you support your body in multiple ways, creating a strong foundation for health and well-being (Lakeside Leisure Centre 2024).

When it comes to exercise, balance and consistency are central. You should find a sustainable routine that fits your physical condition and lifestyle. Aim for a combination of moderate and vigorous activities three to five times throughout the week to keep things interesting and effective. **The American Heart Association recommends at least 150 minutes of moderate aerobic exercise or 75 minutes of vigorous activity per week, along with muscle-strengthening activities on two or more days** (American Heart Association 2025). This might sound like a lot, but it can be broken down into manageable chunks that fit into your schedule. Consistency is more important than intensity, so focus on making exercise a regular habit instead of an occasional hobby.

Small changes can make a big difference. For instance, you might consider taking the stairs instead of the elevator or parking a little farther from your destination to add extra steps to your day. If you work at a desk, set reminders to stand up and stretch or take a short walk every hour. Scheduling regular workout sessions can also help you stay on track—you might try blocking off time in your calendar just as you would for a meeting or appointment. If you are not interested in traditional gym workouts, find activities you enjoy, such as dancing, hiking, or even gardening, which can also provide you with the physical benefits you are looking for.

Advice for Creating a Personal Exercise Plan

Take a moment to write down what types of exercise you enjoy and how you might integrate them into your week. Consider any barriers you might face, like time constraints or lack of motivation, and think about solutions. Could you team up with a friend to make it more fun? Or can you get a group of neighbors together to walk on a regular basis? Perhaps you could explore new classes or activities in your area. Try Tai Chi, chair yoga, or wall Pilates. By creating a personalized exercise plan, you take ownership of your health journey, making it both achievable and enjoyable.

Mindful Eating: Evoking a Healthy Relationship with Food

Mindful eating is a practice that focuses on an individual's sensual awareness of food and their experience of the food (Nelson 2017). Have you ever read a book or newspaper while eating? Did you even notice what you ate? It is important to create a deeper connection with your food and your body's needs. By tuning into hunger and satiety cues, you can better understand when you are actually hungry and when you are satisfied. This awareness helps reduce habits like binge eating or turning to food for emotional comfort. Instead of eating on autopilot, you learn to appreciate your meals, which can lead to healthier eating patterns and improved digestion.

There are several techniques you can use to practice mindful eating. One of the simplest is to eat slowly and

savor each bite. It takes 20 minutes for your body to signal that it is satiated (Blackburn 2018). That means you have continued to eat past the point of satisfying true hunger (Blackburn 2018). By taking your time, you give your body a chance to signal fullness, helping you avoid overeating (Blackburn 2018). It also allows you to enjoy the flavors and textures of your food more fully, turning meals into a pleasurable experience rather than a rushed task. Another effective method is eliminating distractions during meals. This means putting away your phone, turning off the TV, and focusing solely on the act of eating. When you are fully present, you are more likely to listen to your body's cues and make mindful choices.

Being mindful and present during meals can do wonders for your digestion. When you are distracted or stressed while eating, your digestive system does not function as efficiently. Mindful eating encourages you to relax and focus on your food, which can enhance nutrient absorption. When you are calm, your body is better able to break down food and absorb essential vitamins and minerals. This can lead to improved digestive health and reduced bloating or indigestion. By making meals a time of mindfulness, you support your body's natural processes and contribute to overall well-being.

To develop mindful eating practices, start by creating a calm and pleasant dining environment. Set the table, light a candle, or play soft music to create a peaceful atmosphere. Engaging all your senses can also enhance mindfulness. Notice the colors and presentation of your meal, the aroma as you bring it to your mouth, and the textures as you chew. This sensory engagement can make meals more enjoyable and satisfying, reducing the urge to snack mindlessly later. It is also helpful to pause and express gratitude for your food, acknowledging the effort that went into its preparation and its role in nourishing your body. These small steps can transform your eating habits and deepen your relationship with food.

Mindful Eating Reflection

Try this exercise: Before your next meal, take a moment to breathe deeply and set an intention to eat mindfully. As you eat, pay attention to how the food looks, smells, and tastes. Do not rush, and enjoy the company you are with. Notice any changes in your hunger and fullness levels. Afterward, write down your observations in a journal. Reflect on how this experience differed from your usual meals and any insights you gained. This practice can help reinforce the benefits of mindful eating and encourage you to continue exploring this approach.

Stress Management Techniques: Reducing Inflammatory Responses

Stress is more than just a mental burden; it is also a biological response that can have significant effects on your body. When you are under stress, your body releases cortisol, a hormone that is part of the "fight or flight" response (LeWine 2024). While this is a natural reaction, chronic stress can keep cortisol levels elevated, leading to inflammation over time (LeWine 2024). This persistent state of alertness can trigger inflammation by altering immune responses and increasing the production of inflammatory cytokines. If left unchecked, this can contribute to various health issues, from digestive problems to cardiovascular diseases. Understanding this link between stress and inflammation emphasizes the importance of managing stress for your health.

To combat the effects of stress, it is necessary to incorporate stress management techniques into your daily

routine. Meditation is a useful tool that helps calm the mind and reduce stress-induced inflammation. By taking just a few minutes each day to focus on your breath and clear your mind, you can lower cortisol levels and promote relaxation. Deep breathing exercises are equally effective. They help activate the parasympathetic nervous system, which counteracts the stress response. Progressive muscle relaxation is another technique that involves tensing and then relaxing each muscle group in your body. This practice helps reduce physical tension and signals to your brain that it is time to relax, further decreasing stress and inflammation (Robinson, Segal, and Smith 2025).

Incorporating stress relief activities into your daily life is imperative for maintaining balance. Taking short breaks during work, even if it is just for a few minutes to stretch or walk around, can reduce stress levels. These pauses, however short, allow your mind to reset and your body to release tension. Engaging in hobbies and leisure activities that you enjoy can also provide a much-needed escape from daily pressures. Whether it is reading, painting, or gardening, these activities allow you to immerse yourself in something pleasurable, reducing stress and promoting a sense of well-being. Taking some "me time" for yourself should become a habit. Overall, finding joy in simple activities helps shift your focus away from stressors, giving your body a chance to recover from their effects.

Creating a personal stress management plan can equip you with the tools needed to handle stress effectively. Start by identifying your personal stress triggers. Is it work deadlines, family responsibilities, or financial worries? By pinpointing what causes your stress, you can develop strategies to tackle these issues head-on. Next, set realistic stress management goals. This could be as simple as dedicating 10 minutes a day to meditation or scheduling a weekly yoga class. Writing down these goals and tracking your progress can provide motivation and clarity. It is also important to establish a routine that incorporates your favorite stress-relief practices so that they become part of your daily life rather than an afterthought.

The Importance of Sleep: Restorative Practices for Health

Waking up each morning feeling refreshed and ready to take on the day may be only a dream right now. This is the power of a good night's sleep, a fundamental pillar of health that gets overlooked far too often. Adequate sleep is also a critical part of reducing inflammation in the body. **During sleep, your body goes into repair mode, working to heal and restore itself. This is when your immune system gets a chance to recalibrate, improving its ability to fight off infections and reduce inflammation.** Research highlights how poor sleep habits can lead to increased levels of inflammatory markers, making quality sleep a necessary component in our quest to keep inflammation at bay (Harvard Health Publishing 2024).

Several factors can impact the quality of your sleep, and understanding these can help you make changes for the better. The environment in which you sleep plays a significant role. A room that is too warm, too bright, or noisy can disrupt your sleep cycle. Creating a cool, dark, and quiet space can enhance your ability to fall and stay asleep. Red walls, a desk with your computer staring back at you, distracting wall decorations, or collectibles all contribute to a chaotic space that is not conducive to relaxation. Your pre-sleep routine is equally important. Do not exercise within three hours of bedtime or eat within two hours of bedtime. Avoid the use of screens within an hour before bed, as they can interfere with your body's natural sleep signals. The blue light emitted by screens can trick your brain into thinking it is still daytime, making it harder to fall asleep (Pacheco and Rehman 2024).

Improving sleep hygiene involves establishing habits that support better sleep. One of the most effective strategies is to maintain a consistent sleep schedule. Going to bed and waking up at the same time each day, even on weekends, helps regulate your body's internal clock. This consistency can make it easier to fall asleep and wake up naturally. Another key habit is creating a relaxing bedtime routine. This could be as simple as reading a book, taking a warm bath, writing in your journal, or doing some gentle stretches before bed. These activities signal to your body that it is time to wind down, preparing you for restful sleep.

Integrating relaxation techniques into your bedtime routine can further promote better sleep. Guided meditation or guided imagery, for instance, involves visualizing calming scenes or experiences, which can help you relax and ease into sleep. Visualization can transport you to a serene beach or a quiet forest, helping to quiet the mind and reduce stress. **Listening to calming music or natural sounds, like ocean waves, rain, or theta waves, can also be incredibly soothing.** These sounds can mask disruptive noises and create a peaceful atmosphere conducive to sleep. Experimenting with these techniques can help you discover what works best for you, making sleep a restorative experience (Nunez 2020).

Building a Support System: Encouragement and Accountability

Creating a robust support system can significantly enhance your health journey. Having emotional support can make all the difference when your own resolution falters. Family and friends play a central role here, as they offer encouragement, listen to your challenges, and celebrate your victories. Their emotional investment in your well-being can boost your motivation and help hold you accountable. This encouragement can reinforce your commitment to your own health goals, therefore making them feel more achievable.

To build a strong support system, begin by connecting with others who share similar health goals. Joining health-focused groups or clubs can provide you with a sense of community and shared purpose. Whether it is a local running club, a yoga class, or an online group dedicated to healthy eating, being part of a community can establish camaraderie and inspiration. Partnering with a workout buddy or mentor can also be beneficial. This person can offer practical advice, share experiences, and help keep you motivated. Having someone to share the journey with can make the process more enjoyable and fulfilling. Mutual accountability can push you to stay on track, especially on days when your motivation wanes.

Online communities and resources offer additional layers of support. In today's digital age, you can connect with like-minded individuals across the globe. Engaging in online forums and social media groups focused on health and wellness can provide valuable insights and encouragement. These platforms allow you to ask questions, share your progress, and learn from others' experiences. They can also be a space for venting frustrations and celebrating successes, making you feel less isolated. The digital world brings together diverse perspectives and ideas, offering you a wealth of information and support at your fingertips. It is a reminder that you are never alone and that others are walking a similar path.

Nurturing supportive relationships is necessary for maintaining a positive and motivating environment. Open communication with your support partners is important. Share your goals, challenges, and victories with them, and encourage them to do the same. This exchange promotes trust and understanding, strengthening your connections. Celebrating small victories together can also reinforce these bonds. Recognizing achievements, no matter how minor they seem, can boost morale and motivation. Whether it is completing a week of workouts or trying a new healthy recipe, acknowledging these milestones reinforces your commitment to your health goals. The small wins often lead to bigger successes, and having a support system to share them with makes the journey more rewarding.

Tracking Your Progress: Setting and Achieving Health Goals

Monitoring your progress is important when it comes to achieving your health goals. It guides your future decisions and shows you where you have been. Keeping track of your habits and patterns increases self-awareness, helping you identify what works and what does not. This awareness can encourage you to make informed choices that align with your objectives. For instance, noticing that you feel more energized on days you drink enough water may encourage you to prioritize hydration. Similarly, recognizing a pattern of late-night snacking might prompt you to adjust your evening routine. Awareness (and your trusty food journal) is the first step toward meaningful change.

Various methods can help you track your progress, and they range from high-tech gadgets to simple pen and paper. **Health apps and digital trackers are popular choices for their convenience and ability to provide instant feedback. These apps often include step counters, food diaries, and mood trackers, offering a comprehensive view of your health journey.** They allow you to set reminders, track your progress, and celebrate milestones, all from the palm of your hand. If you prefer a more personal touch, journaling can be a useful way to document your journey. Writing down your thoughts, feelings, and observations can deepen your understanding of your habits and behaviors. It is a form of self-assessment that encourages reflection and insight, helping you identify patterns and areas for improvement.

Setting realistic and achievable goals is essential for maintaining motivation and momentum. When crafting your goals, consider using the SMART criteria: Specific, Measurable, Achievable, Relevant, and Time-bound (Bell n.d.). This approach improves your ability to reach your goals by encouraging you to define your objectives and set a completion date (Bell n.d.). Instead of a vague goal like "exercise more," define a **specific target** such as "walk for 30 minutes, five times a week." Ensure it is **measurable** by tracking each walk on your calendar. Make it **achievable** by starting with a manageable routine that fits your lifestyle. Keep it **relevant** to your overall health and fitness goals. Finally, set a **time-bound deadline**, such as committing to this routine for 90 days. This structure provides direction, builds confidence, and creates a sense of accomplishment that fuels further progress.

Regular reflection and adjustment are important for staying on track and making meaningful progress. Take time each month to review your goals and assess your progress. Celebrate your achievements, no matter how small, and use them as motivation to keep pushing forward. If you find that certain goals are not working, do not be afraid to adjust them. Flexibility is central to maintaining momentum and guaranteeing that your goals remain aligned with your constantly shifting priorities. Embrace the process of continuous improvement, and remember that each step, no matter how small, brings you closer to your personal goals.

As such, these lifestyle changes are not isolated tasks, but rather, they are part of a holistic approach to well-being. Tracking your progress establishes accountability, understanding, and growth. Through this, you can create a life that aligns with your values and health goals. As you continue on this path, consider how these practices integrate into your daily routine, supporting your journey toward a healthier life. Transitioning from personal goals to broader health strategies, the next chapter will explore the power of anti-inflammatory foods and how they can be seamlessly incorporated into your meals for sustained health benefits.

Chapter 7

Overcoming Challenges and Sustaining Motivation

At some point, you are likely to find yourself at a lively family gathering, surrounded by the aroma of dishes that have been passed down through family generations. The table is laden with mouthwatering options, many of which are not exactly aligned with your current dietary goals. It is a common scene, one that many of us face when trying to maintain healthy eating habits in social settings. Family gatherings, whether it's Thanksgiving dinner or the summer family reunion, with their traditional foods, can be particularly challenging. Dining out with friends can be equally daunting, especially if the restaurant's menu does not cater to your health-focused lifestyle. But make sure not to fret, as **it is possible to overcome these social situations without derailing your diet.**

Maintaining Your Dietary Goals

The first step in maintaining your diet during social events is to come prepared. One effective strategy is to bring a healthy dish to share. This ensures that there is something you can eat and introduces others to your healthy lifestyle. You might consider preparing a quinoa and vegetable salad or a platter of fresh vegetables with hummus. These dishes are delicious and visually appealing, making them a welcome addition to any gathering. When dining out, take a moment to check the restaurant's menu online beforehand. Many establishments now provide detailed nutritional information, making it easier to choose options that align with your goals. If the menu is limited, you can often request modifications to dishes. Most restaurants are happy to accommodate substitutions, such as swapping out fries for a side salad or asking for dressing on the side. **Eating healthy is not about depriving yourself of foods you enjoy, but rather, it is about making healthy choices for the long term.**

Effectively communicating your dietary preferences is another important aspect of staying true to your diet in social settings. When expressing your needs, assertive communication is key. It is important to be clear and confident without coming across as demanding. You might say, "I am focusing on healthier choices right now, so I will pass on the dessert, but thank you!" Framing your dietary choices in a positive light can also help others understand and respect your decisions. For example, if pressed, you can explain how certain foods make you feel better or contribute to your health goals. This approach informs and invites curiosity, allowing you to share your dietary aspirations in a way that is engaging and informative.

Planning and preparation are extremely useful when going to social events. Eating a filling, healthy snack or meal before a big gathering can help you avoid the temptation to overindulge. A quick snack, like an apple with almond butter or a handful of trail mix or granola, can curb your hunger and keep you grounded in your dietary intentions. Going into a social event with a plan will minimize anxiety and help you make mindful choices, allowing you to enjoy the occasion without feeling deprived.

Interactive Element: How to Create an Eating Checklist

Create a checklist of your favorite go-to strategies for staying on track in social settings. Include items like "Bring a healthy dish," "Research the menu," and "Communicate dietary preferences." Keep this checklist handy to reinforce your intentions and remind you of your tools for success. Adding a few personal motivators or affirmations can boost your confidence and commitment to your dietary goals. **By preparing in advance, you empower yourself to manage social situations with ease and enjoy the experience without compromising your health goals.**

Overcoming Plateaus: Strategies for Continued Progress

Hitting a plateau in your health journey is a common experience and nothing to be discouraged by. Most of the time, plateaus occur because the body has adapted to your routine. The human body is incredibly efficient, always seeking balance. When you repeat the same exercises or stick rigidly to a specific diet, your body becomes accustomed to these patterns. This adaptation, while a sign of progress, can lead to feelings of stagnation. Additionally, a lack of variety in both diet and exercise can leave your body yearning for new challenges, as repetitive actions often result in diminishing returns over time.

To break through a plateau, you might think about shaking things up. One effective strategy is to switch up your exercise routine. If you have been doing the same cardio workout, try incorporating strength training or high-intensity interval training (HIIT). These variations can boost your metabolism and engage different muscle groups, reigniting progress. Similarly, adjusting your caloric intake or macronutrient ratios can help. If you have been consuming the same number of calories daily, a slight increase in carbs from vegetables or decrease in carbs from grains might be just what your body needs to kickstart change. Incorporate more protein to support muscle growth and repair, or experiment with reducing carbohydrates overall if your goal is weight loss. These adjustments can help re-energize your metabolism and push you over a plateau (YouFit 2025). Personally, I can move the needle just by giving up bananas. They're starchy and the ripe ones have a lot of sugar, so that little adjustment seems to work for me.

A shift in mindset can also work effectively when it feels like you are stuck. Focus on non-weight-related victories instead of just numbers. Maybe you have noticed improved energy levels, stamina, better sleep, or a newfound love for cooking healthier meals. These achievements are just as important as any number on a scale. Setting new, challenging goals can also keep your journey exciting. You might aim for a new personal best in a workout or try a new physical activity altogether. These goals keep you motivated and provide a fresh perspective on success, helping to maintain momentum even when progress seems slow.

Tracking and reflecting on your habits can provide valuable insights. Keeping a detailed food and exercise journal helps you identify patterns and areas for improvement. Record what you eat, your workout routines, and how you feel daily. This practice can illuminate subtle changes that might have gone unnoticed, offering clues to adjust your approach. Regularly reviewing your progress allows you to celebrate achievements and adjust plans as needed. Reflect on the past month and ask yourself, "What worked well?" and "What could be improved?" These reflections allow you to make informed decisions and continue moving forward.

Progress Reflection Exercise

Take a moment to reflect on your progress by writing down three non-scale victories you have experienced recently. Consider aspects like fewer episodes of digestive upsets, increased energy, improved sleep, mood, or enhanced fitness. Reflect on how these achievements make you feel and how they contribute to your overall well-being. This exercise can shift your focus from what has not changed to what has, reinforcing your commitment to your health journey.

Handling Skepticism: Educating Others About Your Choices

You have just committed to a healthier lifestyle, and you are excited about the changes. But then comes the skepticism, often from those closest to you. Family, friends, or coworkers might question your choices, sometimes out of genuine concern, other times simply due to misunderstanding. It is not uncommon to face doubt or criticism when you make dietary changes, especially if they differ from the norm. A friend might casually comment, "But you have always loved pizza," inviting you to answer honestly by saying something like, "Pizza is great occasionally, but it makes me feel bloated and sleepy when I eat it." Or a coworker might joke, "Are you sure that's enough protein?" Here, you might respond by saying, "I get lots of protein from other foods I eat, and I would be happy to share them with you if you are interested in learning more about how to eat healthily." These remarks can feel discouraging, but they also present opportunities to educate and share your experience with others.

Recently, at a family dinner, I passed on the grilled cauliflower dish that everyone was raving about. One person said, "Why didn't you try the cauliflower? It is healthy, and you claim to eat healthy foods, but don't you like it?" My response was, "I like cauliflower, but it doesn't like me." He pressed on, "What do you mean it doesn't like you? That doesn't make any sense." By now, everyone was paying attention to this exchange, so I calmly looked at him and said, "Because it makes me gassy." He turned red in the face, a few people giggled, and someone laughed and said, "TMI." That was the last time anyone questioned my food choices, and now I do not have to spend a whole meal defending my diet every time we gather.

If you are not comfortable oversharing, as I did, providing credible resources can also help others understand your choices. Offer articles or studies that back up your dietary decisions. You might say, "I found this interesting, credible article that explains why whole foods can reduce inflammation. I can send it to you if you are interested." This shows that your choices are informed and also invites others to learn more on their own terms. Encourage open dialogues rather than debates. Listen actively to the concerns of others, showing that you respect their opinions even if you disagree. By doing so, you create a space for mutual understanding.

Finding common ground can ease tension and establish supportive conversations. Maybe you both value sustainability or have a shared interest in fitness. Highlight these similarities to bridge gaps. You might suggest trying a healthy recipe together or attending a local health-focused event. Surrounding yourself with like-minded individuals can further bolster your resolve.

Seek out support groups or online forums where you can share experiences and gain insights from others on similar paths. These communities provide a sense of belonging and can be a source of encouragement when facing skepticism.

Building a supportive network extends to seeking out health-conscious communities. This does not mean cutting ties with those who do not share your lifestyle, but rather, it means enriching your social circle with people who uplift your health goals. Attend workshops, cooking classes, or fitness events to meet others who prioritize well-being. These interactions can reinforce your commitment and provide fresh perspectives. Remember, handling skepticism is less about convincing others and more about confidently embracing your choices. By educating and engaging with empathy, you strengthen your resolve and inspire others to join you on the path to better health.

Cooking with Confidence: Building Culinary Skills

Cooking is a useful strategy to force you to stick to your dietary goals. When you cook for yourself, you gain control over every ingredient that goes into your meals. This means you can reduce unwanted additives and choose fresh, wholesome ingredients that align with your health objectives. The ability to cook allows you to whip up dishes that are as delicious as they are nutritious, transforming mealtime from a chore into a creative outlet. It is about embracing the joy of cooking while making sure that your meals are tailored to your personal health needs.

Developing basic cooking techniques is an effective starting point, especially if you are new to the kitchen. Mastering knife skills, for instance, can make meal prep more efficient and enjoyable. Knowing how to properly chop, dice, and slice speeds up cooking and improves the presentation of your dishes. **Understanding cooking methods** like roasting and steaming can elevate simple ingredients into flavorful dishes. Roasting enhances the natural sweetness of vegetables, while steaming preserves nutrients, making it ideal for health-conscious cooking. These techniques provide a foundation for endless culinary exploration, allowing you to create a variety of healthy meals.

Venturing beyond the basics, experimentation in the kitchen opens up a world of possibilities. Reimagine your favorite dishes by swapping out less healthy components for more nutritious alternatives. Love pasta? Try zucchini noodles or alternative grain options. Craving something creamy? Use avocado or Greek yogurt instead of heavy cream. My recipe for spinach artichoke dip replaces the full-fat sour cream and mayonnaise with a light and tasty Greek yogurt and avocado mayo. It is as delicious as the full-fat version, and it goes well with all those crunchy veggies on the crudites platter. These small changes can make a significant difference in the nutritional profile of your meals.

Exploring new cuisines is another way to expand your culinary repertoire. When they say "variety is the spice of life," they are talking about the wide range of spices you can use to liven up your favorite dishes. Explore Mediterranean, Asian, or Middle Eastern flavors, each offering unique ingredients and cooking styles that can make your meals exciting and diverse. This creative process enhances your cooking skills and makes sticking to your diet more enjoyable.

To build your culinary skills, consider tapping into different resources that are designed to guide and inspire. Online cooking classes and tutorials can be extremely useful, providing step-by-step instructions and visual demonstrations. These platforms offer flexibility, allowing you to learn at your own pace and revisit lessons as needed. Recipe books focused on healthy cooking also contain new ideas and techniques. Look for cookbooks that emphasize whole foods and balanced meals, offering recipes that are both accessible and inspiring. These resources can help you discover new flavors, develop your skills, and gain increased confidence in the kitchen.

Embracing Variety: Keeping Your Diet Exciting

Eating the same foods day in and day out can lead to boredom and a lack of motivation. More importantly, it can also result in nutritional gaps, as different foods offer different nutrients. By embracing variety, you keep your meals interesting and ensure a wider intake of vitamins, minerals, and antioxidants. Rotating different protein sources, such as chicken, fish, tofu, and beans, can provide a rich array of amino acids and nutrients that support your overall health. This diversity helps prevent monotony and keeps your diet balanced and nourishing.

Incorporating new foods and flavors into your diet is important. Why not introduce unfamiliar ingredients like quinoa, farro, or jackfruit into your meals? These foods bring unique textures and flavors, offering a welcome change from the norm. Experimenting with spices and herbs can also elevate your dishes. You might add turmeric or saffron to rice, cumin to roasted vegetables, or fresh herbs like basil and cilantro to salads. These additions enhance flavor and provide health benefits, as many spices and herbs are rich in antioxidants and anti-inflammatory compounds. Start small, perhaps by trying one new ingredient each week or experimenting with a different cooking technique for a familiar dish. Over time, you will find that these small steps lead to a broader palate, a richer dining experience, and a more balanced diet. This variety will keep your diet exciting and nutritious while also establishing a deeper connection to the food you eat and the cultures it comes from.

Diversifying your meal preparation methods can further enhance your dining experience. Instead of always opting for the stovetop, consider grilling, baking, or stir-frying your vegetables. Each method brings out different flavors and textures, allowing you to enjoy familiar ingredients in new ways. Grilling adds a smoky depth, baking can intensify sweetness, and stir-frying offers a quick, flavorful option with minimal oil. With a little advance meal prep, you can have your choice of quinoa, brown rice, and farro waiting to throw into a pan for a quick fried rice with chicken or shrimp just by adding peas, some shredded carrots, broccoli, maybe edamame, or mushrooms. Whatever is fresh and on hand can make a quick, delicious, nutritious meal.

Celebrating Small Wins: The Key to Long-Term Success

It is often easy to overlook the small wins, but it is these small wins that open up avenues for greater achievements. These small wins are powerful reminders of your progress and perseverance. Celebrating milestones like improved energy levels or a newfound ability to climb stairs without losing your breath can fuel your motivation and keep you on track. Recognizing these achievements can be as simple as taking a moment to reflect on how much better you feel or treating yourself to something special, such as a new book you have been eyeing or an afternoon spent doing something you love. These personal rewards acknowledge your hard work and inspire you to keep going.

The psychological benefits of recognizing success are significant. This recognition is about enhancing your self-efficacy—the belief in your ability to succeed. When you acknowledge your successes, you reinforce a positive self-image and increase your commitment to your goals. This boost in confidence can spill over into other areas of life, encouraging you to take on new challenges with a positive attitude. Each achievement adds a new block, strengthening the foundation and making it easier to reach even higher. The more you recognize your achievements, the more motivated you will be to continue, creating a cycle of success and self-assurance (Cherry 2024).

Keeping a record of your achievements is an effective way to ensure continuous improvement. Maintaining a success journal allows you to document your progress, standing as a tangible reminder of how far you have come. This practice encourages reflection, helping you identify patterns and recognize what strategies work best for you. It is a chance to look back and see the cumulative effect of your efforts, reinforcing the value of persistence. Sharing your achievements with supportive peers can also amplify this sense of accomplishment. Whether it is a close friend, a partner, or a community group, having others celebrate your successes with you can deepen the experience and provide additional motivation to keep pushing forward.

Success Reflection Prompt

Take a few moments to write down three achievements from the past month, big or small. Reflect on how these successes make you feel and what they say about your progress. Consider sharing one of these achievements with a supportive friend or family member. This reflection can reinforce your commitment and highlight the importance of celebrating each step forward. By acknowledging your achievements, you solidify your progress and inspire those around you.

Celebrating small wins is a fundamental aspect of achieving long-term success. By recognizing and appreciating these milestones, you create a positive feedback loop that strengthens your resolve and enhances your overall experience. Each celebration, no matter how small, is a testament to your dedication and resilience. Embrace these moments, for they are the building blocks of your journey toward a healthier, more fulfilling life. As you continue to explore the power of nutrition and lifestyle changes, remember that every step counts. In the final chapter, this book will discuss the culinary delights and nutritional wonders of the Mediterranean lifestyle, offering a blend of flavors and health benefits that will further enrich your health and diet.

Chapter 8

Recipes Inspired by Mediterranean Diets

Mornings set the tone for the day, and what better way to start than with a meal that fuels your body and mind? Breakfast is an opportunity to nourish yourself and prepare for the business of the day ahead. A nutrient-dense breakfast can boost cognitive function, keep energy levels steady, and even improve your mood. As such, this chapter will explore some delicious Mediterranean-inspired breakfasts that are both satisfying and packed with nutrients to kickstart your day.

Breakfasts to Kickstart Your Day

One of the most versatile breakfast options is Mediterranean-style overnight oats. Begin by mixing rolled oats with almond milk, a dash of cinnamon, and a handful of sliced almonds in a jar. Add a scoop of Greek yogurt for creaminess and a teaspoon of honey for natural sweetness. Top with fresh berries like blueberries or strawberries, which are rich in antioxidants. Let the mixture sit in the refrigerator overnight. By morning, you have a grab-and-go breakfast that is both hearty and delicious. The combination of whole grains, healthy fats, and protein guarantees that you will feel fueled. It is also an easy way to incorporate fiber and vitamins into your morning routine without much fuss.

For those who crave something more indulgent but still healthy, Greek yogurt with mixed berries and honey is a perfect choice. Greek yogurt is higher in protein and lower in sugar than other yogurts. It is filled with protein and probiotics, supporting digestion and keeping you satiated. Top it with a medley of fresh berries—blueberries, raspberries, and blackberries work well—and drizzle with a bit of honey if you really crave the added sweetness. This breakfast is quick to prepare and allows you to start the day with energy, offering a balance of taste and nutrition that can keep you going until lunch.

When time is of the essence, avocado toast on whole-grain bread is a quick yet satisfying breakfast. Simply mash a ripe avocado with a pinch of salt and a squeeze of lemon juice, spreading it generously over toasted whole-grain bread. For an extra protein boost, top with a poached egg or sprinkle with pumpkin seeds. This meal is rich in healthy fats, fiber, and essential nutrients, making it a useful option for those hectic mornings when you need something fast and fulfilling. The combination of textures and flavors delights the palate and provides the energy needed to tackle the morning.

Fiber-rich breakfasts are effective for digestion and keeping you full longer. Alternative whole-grain pancakes with fresh fruit are a good way to enjoy a leisurely breakfast. Use almond flour to make the pancakes, adding a scoop of chia seeds for an extra fiber boost. Serve with a generous topping of fresh fruit like bananas or berries and a drizzle of pure maple syrup. Be sure you are not using high fructose corn syrup, which can cause a spike in insulin. This meal will satisfy your sweet cravings and ensure a steady release of energy throughout the morning. The fiber in the whole grains and chia seeds improves digestion and promotes a feeling of fullness, keeping mid-morning hunger at bay.

Chia seed pudding with almond milk is another brilliant option for those seeking a nutrient-packed breakfast. Mix a few tablespoons of chia seeds with almond milk in a bowl, add a splash of vanilla extract, and let it sit overnight in the fridge. By morning, you will have a creamy pudding-like consistency. Top with nuts, seeds, or fruit for added flavor and nutrition. This breakfast is rich in omega-3 fatty acids, fiber, and protein, making it a perfect choice for anyone looking to start their day on a healthy note. The simplicity of preparation combined with the nutritional benefits makes chia seed pudding a staple in a balanced diet.

Breakfast Planning Checklist

To help incorporate these breakfast ideas into your routine, expand the breakfast planning checklist portion on the Superfood Weekly Meal Plan in Chapter 5. List each breakfast option and the ingredients needed, then check off each day as you prepare and enjoy these meals. This will help you stay organized and make sure that you have all the necessary components for a healthy start to each day.

Energizing Lunches for Midday Vitality

Let's face it: lunchtime is often a much-needed pause in the day, a chance to recharge and refocus. Choosing a balanced meal is essential to maintaining energy levels and mental clarity. A well-rounded lunch can prevent that dreaded afternoon slump, keeping you sharp and productive. One of my favorite go-to lunches is a quinoa salad with edamame, cucumbers, shredded carrots, and lemon-tahini dressing. Quinoa, a complete protein, offers a satisfying base, while edamame or chickpeas add a hearty dose of fiber and protein to keep hunger at bay. Fresh cucumbers provide a refreshing crunch, carrots are sweet and crisp, and the lemon-tahini dressing ties it all together with its tangy goodness. This dish is delicious and also contains an array of nutrients to sustain you through the afternoon.

If you are in the mood for something handheld and portable, a grilled vegetable and hummus wrap might be just what you need. Roasted peppers, zucchini, and eggplant add a robust flavor profile, while a generous spread of hummus provides creaminess and a protein boost. Wrap it all up in a whole-grain or almond flour tortilla, and you have a meal that is easy to pack and carry, perfect for a busy day at work or on the go. This wrap is convenient and a great way to get your veggies in, making it a fantastic option for a nutrient-dense lunch. You can make a variety of hummus flavors by adding Tajin, roasted garlic, roasted red peppers, or avocado and lime to your chickpeas when you blend them up. Use the hummus on breakfast toast, lunch veggie wraps, or as a dip with fresh veggie bites in the afternoon or as a dinner appetizer.

For a meal that is easy to prepare and pack for school or work, you might consider a Mediterranean pasta salad with olives and feta cheese. This salad combines alternative grain pasta, which offers sustained energy, with the tangy flavors of feta and kalamata olives, rich in healthy fats. Toss in cherry tomatoes, red onion, and a sprinkle of fresh basil for a burst of freshness. This dish is ideal for advance meal prep, as the flavors meld beautifully overnight in the fridge, making it even more delicious the next day. It is a colorful, tasty option that can be enjoyed cold or at room temperature, making it versatile and ready whenever you are.

Lentil soup, seasoned with fresh parsley and cumin, is another excellent choice for a nourishing lunch. Lentils are full of protein and fiber, keeping you full and satisfied. The cumin adds a warm, earthy flavor, while the fresh parsley brightens the dish with its subtle peppery notes. This soup is easy to make in large batches, and it stores well, making it a practical choice for lunch throughout the week. Serve it with a slice of Ezekiel bread to round out the meal, and you have a comforting, hearty lunch that is as good for your body as it is for your taste buds.

You might also consider making one of the following lunch bowls:

- Lentils, quinoa, roasted beets, carrots, olive oil, avocado, and chia seeds mixed together in a bowl.
- Farro, roasted vegetables, shredded carrots, radishes, edamame, and dried cranberries mixed together in a bowl.
- Brown rice, chickpeas, leafy super greens, cucumber, olive oil, avocado, and pumpkin seeds mixed together in a bowl.
- Baked sweet potato, dates, almond nut butter, radicchio, and chopped nuts mixed together in a bowl.
- Fava beans, soba noodles, sauteed spinach, quinoa, lightly grilled asparagus, sliced radishes, and avocado oil mixed together in a bowl.
- Brown rice noodles, tofu, edamame, broccoli, and mushrooms (no msg) mixed together in a bowl.
- Vegetable Soup with your favorite veggies mixed together in a bowl.

You might try adding tofu to any bowl for extra protein. Tofu doesn't actually have a flavor of its own and easily picks up the flavor of anything you pair it with like miso, cilantro/lime with garlic and olive oil, or spicy sriracha mayo.

Personally, my biggest meal of the day is lunch. My favorite lunch is a fresh kale salad bowl with beets, dried cranberries, walnuts, and a grilled salmon filet dressed with olive oil and balsamic vinegar. Sometimes, I add shaved brussels sprouts or avocado just to change it up, but I really never get tired of this lunch dish.

Lunchtime Flavor Exploration

Consider keeping a journal to explore different flavor combinations in your lunches. Note which herbs and spices you enjoy most and how they affect the overall taste and satisfaction of your meals. Reflect on how these flavors contribute to your energy and productivity throughout the day. This exercise can help you personalize your lunches to make sure that they are both enjoyable and effective in keeping you energized.

Satisfying Dinners for Health and Happiness

Dinners are a time to unwind, gather with loved ones, and nourish your body. A balanced evening meal brings a sense of closure to the day, allowing you to relax while savoring delicious and wholesome foods. It is an opportunity to connect with family or friends, sharing stories over a table filled with delicious food. Dinner should be a calming ritual, one that provides essential nutrients and satisfies your palate, setting the stage for a restful night ahead. The Mediterranean approach to dinner emphasizes this balance, focusing on lean proteins, whole grains, and fresh ingredients that support both health and happiness (Dominguez 2024).

One delightful dish that embodies this philosophy is baked or grilled salmon with dill and lemon, served alongside quinoa or farro. Salmon, rich in omega-3 fatty acids, supports heart health and reduces inflammation. Baking it with a sprinkle of dill and a squeeze of lemon enhances its natural flavors while also preserving its nutrients. Pair it with quinoa for extra protein or farro, an ancient grain known for its chewy texture and nutty taste. Farro is packed with fiber, which enhances digestion and keeps you satisfied. This combination provides a hearty dose of nutrients that make for a fulfilling dinner.

For those nights when you crave something comforting but still nutritious, you might consider stuffed bell peppers with quinoa and edamame or black beans. The peppers are filled with a savory mixture of quinoa, beans, diced tomatoes, and aromatic spices. This plant-based meal is full of protein and fiber, offering a satisfying and healthy alternative to meat-based dishes. Quinoa blends seamlessly with the creamy texture of the beans, creating a filling that is both hearty and light. The spices add a depth of flavor, turning a simple dish into a culinary experience. It is perfect for anyone looking to reduce meat consumption without sacrificing taste or nutrition.

Eggplant moussaka with a chickpea crust is another delicious vegetarian option. This dish is a Mediterranean classic, reimagined for those who prefer plant-based meals. Layers of roasted eggplant are combined with a rich tomato sauce seasoned with herbs like oregano and thyme. The chickpea crust adds a unique twist, providing a crispy texture that complements the softness of the eggplant. Chickpeas are a good source of protein and fiber, making this dish both nutritious and satisfying. This moussaka is a beautiful blend of flavors and textures, resulting in a comforting meal that is perfect for any evening.

Traditional Mediterranean cooking techniques play a central role in preserving flavors and nutrients. One such method is slow cooking, which allows ingredients to meld together over time, creating rich and complex dishes. Slow-cooked lamb with rosemary and garlic is a prime example. The lamb, seasoned with fresh rosemary and garlic, is cooked slowly until it becomes tender and flavorful. This method allows the natural juices to infuse the meat, enhancing its taste while retaining its nutritional value. Serve it with roasted vegetables or a simple salad for a meal that is both elegant and nourishing. Slow cooking elevates the flavors and makes the preparation process more manageable, as you can set it and forget it.

You might tweak and diversify the above dishes to include different types of protein, legumes and grains, vegetables, and nuts and seeds. Here are some options I recommend:

- **Protein:** Grilled or baked Fish, shellfish, Chicken, Turkey, and/or Tofu.
- **Legumes and Grains:** lentils, beans, farro, quinoa, and/or chickpeas.
- **Fresh, Roasted or Sauteed Vegetables**
- **Nuts and Seeds:** Almonds, walnuts, cashews, brazil nuts, and/or pine nuts.

These dinner ideas are invitations to explore the joys of cooking and eating. Whether you are cooking for yourself or sharing a meal with others, these Mediterranean-inspired recipes offer a path to health and happiness, one delicious bite at a time.

Snacks and Sides: Small Bites with Big Benefits

Snacks and sides might not be considered central to the dining table, but they play an important role in maintaining a balanced diet. They bridge the gap between meals, keep energy levels stable, and help curb overeating at main meals by maintaining satiety.

Here are some suggestions for snacking effectively:

- **Foods you can eat consistently:** Fruit, vegetables, legumes, nuts, seeds, healthy fats, vinegars, and all of your favorite herbs and spices.
- **Foods you should eat in moderation when snacking (2 to 3 times per week):** Meat, seafood, dairy, eggs, and pecorino cheese.
- **Drinks you can consume consistently:** Calorie-free beverages, water, herbal and unsweetened teas, black coffee, and occasionally (once a week) wine.
- **Food and drink you should avoid when snacking:** Red and processed meat, white sugar, refined grains, processed foods, butter, and alcohol.

More specifically, roasted chickpeas with smoked paprika are a prime snack that is both crunchy and flavorful. Chickpeas contain protein and fiber, making them a satisfying choice for keeping hunger at bay. To prepare, simply toss canned chickpeas with olive oil, smoked paprika, and a pinch of salt, then roast them at 400 degrees (F) for 20 to 35 minutes until crispy. The result is a snack with a smoky kick that you can enjoy guilt-free. Whether eaten by the handful or sprinkled over salads for a bit of crunch, roasted chickpeas are versatile and easy to make. They are great for those moments when you need a quick energy boost.

Similarly, grilled zucchini with lemon and mint is a light, refreshing side that pairs well with a variety of main courses. Slice the zucchini lengthwise, brush with olive oil, and grill 3 or 4 minutes until tender. A squeeze of lemon juice and a sprinkle of fresh mint leaves brighten the flavors, creating a side dish that is both vibrant and nutritious. This dish adds a pop of color to your plate and provides vitamins and minerals that support overall health.

Another side dish that is easy to prepare is a tomato and cucumber salad with basil vinaigrette. Fresh tomatoes and cucumbers are sliced or diced and tossed with a simple dressing of olive oil, balsamic vinegar, and fresh basil. The result is a salad that is crisp, tangy, and full of Mediterranean flavors. It is a complement to grilled meats or can be enjoyed on its own for a light meal. The combination of fresh vegetables and herbs enhances the taste and boosts the nutritional value.

Additionally, olives are a staple in Mediterranean diets, known for their healthy fats and antioxidant properties. A homemade tapenade made from olives, capers, and a touch of garlic can transform a piece of whole-grain bread into a sophisticated snack. This spread captures the essence of Mediterranean cuisine, offering depth of flavor and a nutrient boost. It is about enjoying flavors that have stood the test of time and contributed to the well-being of generations.

Sweet Treats: Enjoying Desserts Without Guilt

Desserts can often feel like a guilty pleasure. However, there is no reason they cannot be nourishing and enjoyable. Embracing healthy desserts allows you to satisfy your sweet cravings without compromising your health. It is all about choosing the right ingredients, ones that provide sweetness alongside nutrients.

Now, think of the comforting aroma of baked apples with cinnamon and raisins wafting through your kitchen. Apples, when baked, turn soft and sweet, releasing their natural sugars. Combined with the warmth of cinnamon—a spice known for its anti-inflammatory properties—this dessert becomes a symphony of flavors. Sprinkle in some raisins for added sweetness and fiber. Baking these ingredients together caramelizes the apples and creates a comforting dish that feels like a warm hug on a chilly day. It is a dessert that invites you to savor each bite slowly, appreciating the natural sweetness and the simple pleasures of wholesome ingredients.

For those who crave a bit of decadence, almond flour cookies with dark chocolate chips offer a delicious solution. Almond flour has a light, nutty flavor and is a fantastic gluten-free alternative to traditional wheat flour. It's high in protein and healthy fats, making it a more nutritious option. Dark chocolate chips provide a hit of antioxidants and a deep, satisfying cocoa flavor. These cookies are a testament to the idea that indulgence does not have to mean compromise. Each bite is a balance of sweet and nutty, with a texture that melts in your mouth. Enjoying these cookies is about appreciating the quality of the ingredients and the love put into making them.

Moderation is necessary when it comes to enjoying sweets. This is focused on savoring each bite and allowing the flavors to linger instead of rushing through in one quick gulp. Mindful indulgence means being present with your dessert, recognizing it as a treat rather than a staple. This approach helps you appreciate the dessert fully, leaving you satisfied with less. Consider serving smaller portions or using smaller plates, which can make a dessert feel more abundant. Pairing desserts with a cup of herbal tea or a glass of fruit-flavored water can also slow down the eating process, enhancing overall enjoyment.

Dessert Serving Size Guide

Creating a visual guide to dessert serving sizes can help you practice moderation. Use ice cream scoops in one-, two-, four-, and five-ounce sizes to make portions easier. A five-ounce scoop of farro, quinoa, brown rice, or barley makes a perfect base for a bowl salad, or for sorbets, berries, and frozen yogurt, you get a heart-healthy serving of a sweet treat. By visually seeing the recommended portion sizes for different desserts, you can enjoy your treats without overindulging. This guide can serve as a helpful reminder that quality over quantity is key when it comes to indulgence (Schervish 2018).

Beverages and Smoothies: Refreshing and Nutritious Options

Staying hydrated is necessary for overall health, but it often gets overlooked (Healthdirect 2023). If you are not a fan of plain water, add a squeeze of lemon or other unsweetened fruit juice. Beverages can do more than just quench your thirst; they can also be a vehicle for essential nutrients. When thoughtfully chosen, drinks can enhance your diet, replenish electrolytes, and even provide a moment of relaxation. There is something inherently satisfying about sipping on a refreshing drink that cools you down and contributes to your well-being. Infused waters, for example, are an easy way to add a hint of flavor without any added sugars or artificial ingredients. Cucumber and mint-infused water is a classic choice. Simply slice a fresh cucumber, add a few sprigs of mint, and let them mingle in a pitcher of water in the fridge. This drink is both refreshing and hydrating, offering a gentle detox to your system. The cucumber provides a crispness, while the mint adds a cool, invigorating taste, making it a perfect summertime thirst-quencher.

Herbal teas are another great option. My favorites include hibiscus, mango ginger, or pomegranate/green tea. They can be enjoyed hot or cold, providing a comforting ritual that can soothe or energize. A classic combination like lemon and ginger tea offers a burst of flavor while supporting digestion. Ginger is known for its anti-inflammatory properties, and lemon adds a zesty brightness that is both uplifting and refreshing (Wartenberg 2023). If you can't find this combination in a ready tea bag, just steep fresh ginger root slices in hot water, add a squeeze of lemon, and voila. Or make a quart of your favorite flavor and put it in the fridge to enjoy all day. It is a simple concoction that can be adapted to suit your taste, whether you prefer it stronger or milder.

Of course, smoothies deserve a spotlight as well. If you generally do not enjoy eating breakfast but want to kickstart your metabolism in the morning, a smoothie is an effective way to pack in fruits, vegetables, and healthy fats, making them ideal for breakfast or a nutritious snack. A green smoothie with spinach, avocado, and banana is full of nutrients. Spinach provides iron and fiber without altering the taste, while avocado adds creaminess and healthy fats that promote satiety. Banana brings natural sweetness and potassium, creating a balanced blend that tastes as good as it feels (Aldeborgh 2024).

Mediterranean ingredients can also elevate your beverage game. Pomegranate juice, for example, is a staple in many Mediterranean diets, celebrated for its high antioxidant content. A splash of lime juice can enhance the flavor, adding a tart, refreshing note that complements the sweetness of the pomegranate. This combination delights the palate, supports heart health, and reduces inflammation. It is an easy way to incorporate traditional flavors into your daily routine, connecting you to a rich culinary heritage while nourishing your body.

Infused Water Inspiration Chart

Citrus Infusions

Base	Herb/ Spice	Optional Add-in	Benefits
Lemon + Orange	Basil	Cucumber	Digestive aid, vitamin C boost
Lime + Grapefruit	Mint	Strawberry	Metabolism boost, refreshing
Lemon + Lime	Rosemary	Blueberry	Antioxidant rich, immune support
Orange + Tangerine	Thyme	Raspberry	Vitamin C, mood lifting
Blood Orange	Lavender	Blackberry	Calming, antioxidant rich

Berry Bliss

Base	Herb/ Spice	Optional Add-in	Benefits
Strawberry	Basil	Lemon	Heart health, anti-inflammatory
Blueberry	Mint	Lime	Brain health, antioxidant
Raspberry	Sage	Orange	Digestive aid, vitamin rich
Blackberry	Rosemary	Ginger	Immunity boost, digestive health
Mixed Berries	Thyme	Cucumber	Detoxifying, antioxidant rich

Garden Fresh

Base	Herb/ Spice	Optional Add-in	Benefits
Cucumber	Mint	Lime	Hydrating, cooling
Celery	Cilantro	Lemon	Detoxifying, alkalizing
Cucumber	Dill	Strawberry	Digestive aid, refreshing
Bell Pepper	Basil	Orange	Vitamin rich, metabolism boost
Tomato	Thyme	Lime	Antioxidant rich, heart health

Tropical Escapes

Base	Herb/ Spice	Optional Add-in	Benefits
Pineapple	Mint	Coconut Water	Digestive enzyme boost, hydrating
Mango	Cilantro	Lime	Vitamin A rich, immunity boost
Watermelon	Basil	Strawberry	Hydrating, antioxidant rich
Kiwi	Mint	Cucumber	Vitamin C boost, digestive aid
Passion Fruit	Lemongrass	Orange	Immunity boost, calming

Spice & Everything Nice

Base	Herb/ Spice	Optional Add-in	Benefits
Apple	Cinnamon	Lemon	Metabolism boost, blood sugar balance
Pear	Star Anise	Vanilla Bean	Digestive aid, soothing
Cherry	Cardamom	Lime	Anti-inflammatory, antioxidant
Peach	Clove	Ginger	Immunity boost, digestive aid
Plum	Nutmeg	Orange	Antioxidant rich, calming

Preparation Tips:

- Use filtered water for best flavor
- Muddle herbs gently to release oils
- Allow to infuse for at least 2 hours (4+ hours for best flavor)
- Keep refrigerated for up to 3 days
- Use organic produce when possible
- For stronger flavor, freeze fruit before infusing

Here's an infusion inspiration chart, listing various combinations of fruits, herbs, and spices for your infused waters. This visual guide can spark ideas and encourage creativity, making it easier to enjoy a variety of flavors and keep hydration interesting.

As you explore these beverages and smoothies, remember that they are a way to nourish both body and spirit. Whether you are reaching for a glass of infused water during a hot day or relaxing with a cup of herbal tea in the evening, each sip is a step toward better health.

Incorporating Blue Zone and Mediterranean-inspired meals into your daily routine is a simple yet powerful way to nourish your body while embracing vibrant, wholesome flavors. From nutrient-dense breakfasts that set the tone for the day to satisfying lunches, hearty dinners, and guilt-free desserts, each meal presents an opportunity to fuel yourself with ingredients that promote longevity and well-being. By prioritizing whole foods, healthy fats, and mindful eating, you can enjoy the benefits of sustained energy, improved digestion, and overall vitality.

Breakfast - 10 Anti-Inflammatory Mediterranean & Blue Zone Inspired Recipes

Egg-Based Breakfasts

1. Mediterranean Vegetable Frittata

Serving Size: 2 (½ frittata serving)
Calories: Approximately 290 calories each

Ingredients:

- 6 eggs
- 1 cup spinach, whole leaf or rough chopped
- ½ cup cherry tomatoes, halved
- ¼ cup red bell pepper, diced
- 2 tablespoons olive oil
- 1 small onion, diced
- 2 cloves garlic, minced
- ¼ cup feta cheese (optional)
- 1 teaspoon dried oregano
- Fresh basil leaves
- Salt and pepper to taste

Instructions:

1. Preheat oven to 375°F (190°C).
2. Heat olive oil in an oven-safe skillet over medium heat.
3. Sauté onion until translucent, about 3 minutes.
4. Add garlic, bell pepper, and cook for 2 minutes.
5. Add spinach and tomatoes, cook until spinach wilts.
6. Whisk eggs in a bowl with salt, pepper, and oregano.

7. Pour egg mixture over vegetables in the skillet.
8. Cook until edges begin to set, about 3-4 minutes.
9. Sprinkle with feta if using.
10. Transfer skillet to oven and bake for 10-12 minutes until set.
11. Garnish with fresh basil before serving.

2. Turmeric Scrambled Eggs with Avocado Toast

Serving Size: 1
Calories: Approximately 380 calories

Ingredients:

- 2 eggs
- ½ teaspoon ground turmeric
- ¼ teaspoon ground ginger
- Pinch of black pepper
- 1 tablespoon olive oil
- 1 slice whole grain bread
- ½ avocado
- 1 tablespoon pumpkin seeds
- Red pepper flakes (optional)
- Fresh cilantro for garnish
- Salt to taste

Instructions:

1. Whisk eggs with turmeric, ginger, salt, and pepper.
2. Heat olive oil in a non-stick pan over medium-low heat.
3. Pour in egg mixture and stir gently until soft curds form.
4. Meanwhile, toast the bread.
5. Mash avocado with a fork and spread on toast.

6. Top avocado toast with scrambled eggs.
7. Sprinkle with pumpkin seeds, red pepper flakes, and cilantro.

To save 75 calories and lower cholesterol level use 1 egg

3. Greek Yogurt Breakfast Bowl with Soft-Boiled Eggs

Serving Size: 1
Calories: Approximately 320 calories

Ingredients:

- 2 eggs
- 1 cup Greek yogurt
- 1 tablespoon olive oil
- 1 teaspoon za'atar spice blend
- ¼ cup cucumber, diced
- ¼ cup cherry tomatoes, halved
- 2 tablespoons pitted Kalamata olives, chopped
- 1 tablespoon hemp seeds
- Fresh dill and mint leaves
- Salt and pepper to taste

Instructions:

1. Put 2 eggs in a small pot of water and bring to a boil. Cook for 6½ minutes.
2. Transfer eggs to an ice bath, then peel.
3. Spread Greek yogurt in a shallow bowl.
4. Drizzle with olive oil and sprinkle with za'atar.
5. Arrange cucumber, tomatoes, and olives around the bowl.

6. Cut eggs in half and place on top.
7. Top with hemp seeds, fresh herbs, salt, and pepper.

To save 75 calories and lower cholesterol level use 1 egg

Za'atar spice blend in a combination of herbs like thyme, oregano, marjoram, toasted sesame seeds and sumac (dried ground berries of the sumac plant has a tangy, lemony flavor and bright purple red color)

4. Shakshuka with Swiss Chard and Chickpeas

Serving Size: 2 (2 eggs each)
Calories: Approximately 350 calories

Ingredients:

- 4 eggs
- 1 bunch Swiss chard, stems removed and leaves chopped
- 1 can (15 oz) diced tomatoes
- ½ cup cooked chickpeas
- 1 onion, diced
- 2 cloves garlic, minced
- 1 red bell pepper, diced
- 2 tablespoons olive oil
- 1 teaspoon ground cumin
- 1 teaspoon paprika
- ½ teaspoon turmeric
- Pinch of cayenne pepper (optional)
- Fresh parsley for garnish
- Salt and pepper to taste

Instructions:

1. Heat olive oil in a large skillet over medium heat.
2. Add onion and bell pepper, sauté until softened, about 5 minutes.
3. Add garlic, cumin, paprika, turmeric, and cayenne (if using), cook for 1 minute.
4. Add diced tomatoes, chickpeas, and Swiss chard.
5. Simmer until sauce thickens slightly, about 5-8 minutes.
6. Make 4 wells in the sauce and crack an egg into each.
7. Cover and cook until eggs are set, about 5-7 minutes.
8. Garnish with fresh parsley before serving.

To save 75 calories and lower cholesterol level use 1 egg per serving

Swiss chard stems can be sliced, like celery, and used in soups or veggie stir fries.

5. Sweet Potato and Kale Breakfast Hash with Fried Eggs

Serving Size: 2 (1 egg each)
Calories: Approximately 310

Ingredients:

- 2 eggs
- 1 medium sweet potato, diced
- 2 cups kale, chopped
- ½ onion, diced
- 1 clove garlic, minced
- 2 tablespoons olive oil

- 1 teaspoon smoked paprika
- ½ teaspoon turmeric
- 1 tablespoon fresh rosemary, chopped
- 2 tablespoons walnuts, chopped
- Salt and pepper to taste

Instructions:

1. Heat 1 tablespoon olive oil in a skillet over medium heat.
2. Add sweet potato and cook until beginning to soften, about 5-10 minutes.
3. Add onion and cook for 3 more minutes.
4. Add garlic, paprika, turmeric, salt, and pepper, cook for 1 minute.
5. Add kale and rosemary, cook until kale wilts and sweet potatoes are tender.
6. In a separate pan, heat remaining olive oil over medium-low heat.
7. Fry eggs to your preference.
8. Serve hash topped with fried eggs and sprinkled with walnuts.

For kale, remove spines and double rinse leaves to reduce bitterness

Egg-Free Breakfasts

6. Blueberry Almond Overnight Oats

Serving Size: 1
Calories: Approximately 290 calories

Ingredients:

- ½ cup rolled oats
- ½ cup almond milk
- ¼ cup Greek yogurt
- 1 tablespoon chia seeds
- ½ cup blueberries
- 2 tablespoons chopped or slivered almonds
- 1 tablespoon flax seeds (fresh ground)
- ½ teaspoon cinnamon
- 1 teaspoon honey or maple syrup (optional)
- Fresh mint leaves for garnish

Instructions:

1. In a jar or container, combine oats, almond milk, yogurt, chia seeds, and cinnamon.
2. Stir well, cover, and refrigerate overnight.
3. In the morning, top with blueberries, almonds, flax seeds, and honey if using.
4. Garnish with fresh mint leaves.

7. Mediterranean Quinoa Breakfast Bowl

Serving Size: 1
Calories: Approximately 340 calories

Ingredients:

- ½ cup cooked quinoa
- ¼ cup pomegranate seeds
- ¼ cup pistachios, chopped
- ½ apple, diced

- 2 dried figs, chopped
- 2 tablespoons coconut flakes
- ½ teaspoon cinnamon
- ¼ teaspoon cardamom
- ½ cup almond milk
- 1 teaspoon honey (optional)

Instructions:

1. Warm cooked quinoa with almond milk in a small saucepan.
2. Stir in cinnamon and cardamom.
3. Transfer to a bowl and top with pomegranate seeds, pistachios, apple, figs, and coconut flakes.
4. Drizzle with honey if desired.

8. Sardine and Avocado Toast with Microgreens

Serving Size: 1 serving (2 slices of toast)
Calories: Approximately 400 calories

Ingredients:

- 2 slices whole grain or sprouted Ezekiel bread
- 1 can sardines in olive oil, drained
- 1 small avocado, mashed
- 1 tablespoon lemon juice
- 1 cup microgreens or arugula
- 1 tablespoon olive oil
- 1 teaspoon hemp seeds
- Red pepper flakes
- Salt and black pepper to taste

Instructions:

1. Toast bread slices.
2. Mix mashed avocado with lemon juice, salt, and pepper.
3. Spread avocado mixture on toast.
4. Top with sardines.
5. In a small bowl, toss microgreens with olive oil and a pinch of salt.
6. Place dressed microgreens on top of sardines.
7. Sprinkle with hemp seeds and red pepper flakes.

9. Berry and Kale Smoothie Bowl

Serving Size: 1
Calories: Approximately 270 calories

Ingredients:

- 1 cup mixed berries (blueberries, strawberries, raspberries)
- 1 cup kale leaves, stems removed
- ½ banana
- ¼ avocado
- ¼ cup Greek yogurt
- ½ cup almond milk
- 1 tablespoon ground flax seeds
- **Toppings:**
    - 1 tablespoon pumpkin seeds
    - 1 tablespoon unsweetened coconut flakes
    - 1 tablespoon goji berries
    - ½ kiwi, sliced
    - 1 teaspoon bee pollen (optional)

Instructions:

1. Blend berries, kale, banana, avocado, yogurt, almond milk, and flax seeds until smooth.
2. Pour into a bowl.
3. Arrange toppings decoratively on the surface.
4. Serve immediately.

10. Warm Farro Breakfast Bowl with Figs and Walnuts

Serving Size: 1
Calories: Approximately 380 calories

Ingredients:

- ½ cup cooked farro
- 1 tablespoon olive oil
- ¼ cup walnuts, chopped
- 2 dried figs, chopped
- 2 dates, pitted and chopped
- ½ apple, diced
- ½ teaspoon cinnamon
- ¼ teaspoon nutmeg
- ½ cup almond milk
- 1 tablespoon maple syrup (optional)
- 1 tablespoon fresh mint, chopped

Instructions:

1. In a small saucepan, combine cooked farro and almond milk.
2. Heat over medium-low heat until warm.
3. Stir in cinnamon, nutmeg, and maple syrup if using.

4. Transfer to a bowl and drizzle with olive oil.
5. Top with walnuts, figs, dates, and apples.
6. Garnish with fresh mint.

Lunch - 10 Anti-Inflammatory Mediterranean & Blue Zone Inspired Recipes

Protein-Based Lunches (Fish, Chicken, Eggs)

1. Mediterranean Herb-Baked Salmon with Quinoa Tabbouleh

Servings: 1
Calories: Approximately 450 calories

Ingredients:

- 4 oz salmon fillet
- 2 tablespoons olive oil, divided
- 1 tablespoon fresh lemon juice
- 2 cloves garlic, minced
- 1 teaspoon dried oregano
- ½ cup cooked quinoa
- ¼ cup cherry tomatoes, quartered
- ¼ cup cucumber, diced
- 2 tablespoons red onion, finely diced
- ¼ cup fresh parsley, chopped
- 2 tablespoons fresh mint, chopped
- 1 tablespoon hemp seeds
- Salt and pepper to taste

Instructions:

1. Preheat the oven to 375°F (190°C).
2. Mix 1 tablespoon olive oil with lemon juice, garlic, oregano, salt, and pepper.
3. Place salmon on a baking sheet and brush with olive oil herb mixture. You can sear the skin side of the salmon in olive oil first if you prefer.
4. Bake for 12-15 minutes until the salmon flakes easily.
5. Meanwhile, in a bowl, combine quinoa, tomatoes, cucumber, red onion, parsley, and mint. You can also use extra fine bulgur instead of quinoa.
6. Dress tabbouleh with remaining olive oil, salt, and pepper.
7. Serve salmon on a bed of quinoa tabbouleh and sprinkle with hemp seeds.

2. Turmeric Chicken with Roasted Sweet Potatoes and Broccoli

Servings: 1
Calories: Approximately 380 calories

Ingredients:

- 4 oz chicken breast
- 1 teaspoon turmeric
- ½ teaspoon ground ginger
- ¼ teaspoon black pepper
- 1 tablespoon olive oil
- 1 small sweet potato, cubed
- 1 cup broccoli florets
- 1 teaspoon garlic powder

- 1 tablespoon fresh rosemary, chopped
- 2 tablespoons walnuts, chopped
- Salt to taste

Instructions:

1. Preheat the oven to 400°F (200°C).
2. Mix turmeric, ginger, black pepper, and salt.
3. Rub chicken breast with spice mixture and 1 teaspoon olive oil.
4. On a baking sheet, toss sweet potatoes and broccoli with remaining olive oil, garlic powder, rosemary, and salt.
5. Place chicken on the same baking sheet.
6. Roast for 20-25 minutes, until chicken is cooked through and vegetables are tender. Chicken must reach 165 degrees (F) minimum internal temperature.
7. Sprinkle roasted vegetables with chopped walnuts before serving.

3. Greek Power Bowl with Sardines and Farro

Servings: 1
Calories: Approximately 420 calories

Ingredients:

- 1 can sardines in olive oil, drained
- ½ cup cooked farro or quinoa
- 1 cup fresh arugula
- ½ cup cherry tomatoes, halved
- ¼ cup cucumber, diced
- 2 tablespoons red onion, thinly sliced
- 2 tablespoons Kalamata olives, pitted and halved

- 2 tablespoons feta cheese (optional)
- 1 tablespoon fresh lemon juice
- 1 tablespoon olive oil
- 1 teaspoon dried oregano
- 1 tablespoon pine nuts, fresh or lightly toasted
- Salt and pepper to taste

Instructions:

1. In a bowl, arrange arugula as the base.
2. Top with cooked farro, sardines, tomatoes, cucumber, red onion, and olives.
3. In a small bowl, whisk together lemon juice, olive oil, oregano, salt, and pepper.
4. Drizzle dressing over the bowl.
5. Sprinkle with feta cheese (if using) and pine nuts.

4. Spinach and Mushroom Frittata with Avocado Salad

Servings: 2
Calories: Approximately 340 calories per serving

Ingredients:

- 3 eggs, beaten
- 1 cup spinach, chopped
- ½ cup mushrooms, sliced
- 1 small onion, diced
- 1 clove garlic, minced
- 1 tablespoon olive oil
- 1 teaspoon dried thyme
- ½ avocado, sliced
- 1 cup mixed greens (arugula, watercress, baby spinach)

- ½ cup cherry tomatoes, halved
- 1 tablespoon balsamic vinegar
- Salt and pepper to taste

Instructions:

1. Preheat the oven to 375°F (190°C).
2. Heat olive oil in an oven-safe skillet over medium heat.
3. Sauté onions until translucent, about 3 minutes.
4. Add mushrooms and garlic, cook until mushrooms are lightly browned.
5. Add spinach and cook until wilted.
6. Pour beaten eggs over vegetables, season with thyme, salt, and pepper.
7. Cook until edges begin to set, then transfer to the oven.
8. Bake for 10-12 minutes until fully set.
9. Meanwhile, toss mixed greens and tomatoes with balsamic vinegar and olive oil.
10. Serve frittata with salad and sliced avocado.

To save 75 calories and lower cholesterol level remove 1 egg

5. Mackerel and White Bean Salad with Lemon-Herb Dressing

Servings: 1
Calories: Approximately 390 calories

Ingredients:

- 4 oz smoked mackerel, flaked
- ½ cup white beans, rinsed and drained
- 2 cups mixed dark leafy greens (kale, spinach, arugula)

- ¼ cup red bell pepper, diced
- 2 tablespoons red onion, thinly sliced
- 1 tablespoon capers
- 1 tablespoon fresh dill, chopped
- 1 tablespoon fresh parsley, chopped
- 2 tablespoons olive oil
- 1 tablespoon lemon juice
- 1 teaspoon Dijon mustard
- 1 small garlic clove, minced
- Salt and pepper to taste

Instructions:

1. In a large bowl, combine greens, bell pepper, red onion, and capers.
2. In a small bowl, whisk together olive oil, lemon juice, Dijon mustard, garlic, salt, and pepper.
3. Drizzle dressing over salad and toss.
4. Gently fold in white beans and flaked mackerel.
5. Garnish with fresh dill and parsley before serving.

Vegetarian/Vegan Lunches

6. Lentil and Vegetable Buddha Bowl with Turmeric Tahini Dressing

Servings: 1
Calories: Approximately 420 calories

Ingredients:

- ½ cup cooked lentils

- 1 cup roasted vegetables (sweet potatoes, broccoli, cauliflower)
- 1 cup shredded kale, massaged with olive oil
- ¼ cup cooked quinoa
- ¼ avocado, sliced
- 2 tablespoons pomegranate seeds
- 1 tablespoon pumpkin seeds

For the dressing:

- 2 tablespoons tahini
- 1 tablespoon lemon juice
- 1 teaspoon turmeric
- ¼ teaspoon ground ginger
- 1 small garlic clove, minced
- 2-3 tablespoons water
- Salt and pepper to taste

Instructions:

1. Arrange kale as the base in a bowl.
2. Add sections of lentils, roasted vegetables, and quinoa.
3. Top with avocado slices, pomegranate seeds, and pumpkin seeds.
4. Whisk together all dressing ingredients until smooth.
5. Drizzle dressing over the bowl before serving.

Remove spines and double rinse kale to reduce bitterness

7. Mediterranean Stuffed Sweet Potatoes with Chickpeas

Servings: 1
Calories: Approximately 360 calories

Ingredients:

- 1 medium sweet potato
- ½ cup cooked or canned chickpeas, rinsed and drained
- ¼ cup cherry tomatoes, quartered
- 2 tablespoons red onion, diced
- 2 tablespoons parsley, chopped
- 1 tablespoon olive oil
- 1 tablespoon lemon juice
- ½ teaspoon ground cumin
- ¼ teaspoon paprika
- 1 tablespoon tahini
- 2 tablespoons plain Greek yogurt (omit for vegan)
- 1 tablespoon pine nuts, fresh or lightly toasted
- Salt and pepper to taste

Instructions:

1. Preheat the oven to 400°F (200°C).
2. Pierce sweet potato several times with a fork or cut into cubes and bake for 45-60 minutes until tender.
3. In a bowl, combine chickpeas, tomatoes, red onion, and parsley.
4. Dress with olive oil, lemon juice, cumin, paprika, salt, and pepper.
5. Split open the baked sweet potato and stuff with chickpea mixture.
6. Drizzle with tahini and top with Greek yogurt (if using).

7. Sprinkle with pine nuts before serving.

8. Warm Farro Salad with Roasted Vegetables and Pistachios

Servings: 1
Calories: Approximately 410 calories

Ingredients:

- ¾ cup cooked farro
- 1 cup mixed roasted vegetables (beets, carrots, Brussels sprouts)
- 2 cups arugula
- 2 tablespoons pistachios, chopped
- 2 dried figs, chopped
- 2 tablespoons olive oil
- 1 tablespoon balsamic vinegar
- 1 teaspoon Dijon mustard
- 1 small shallot, minced
- 1 teaspoon honey (optional, omit for vegan)
- Salt and pepper to taste

Instructions:

1. In a large bowl, combine warm farro with arugula so the greens wilt slightly.
2. Add roasted vegetables and dried figs.
3. In a small bowl, whisk together olive oil, balsamic vinegar, Dijon mustard, shallot, honey (if using), salt, and pepper.
4. Toss salad with dressing.
5. Top with chopped pistachios before serving.

9. Tofu and Vegetable Stir-Fry with Ginger-Turmeric Sauce

Servings: 1
Calories: Approximately 330 calories

Ingredients:

- 4 oz firm tofu
- 1 cup broccoli florets
- ½ cup red bell pepper, sliced
- ½ cup carrots, julienned
- ½ cup mushrooms, sliced
- 2 cloves garlic, minced
- 1 tablespoon fresh ginger, grated
- 2 tablespoons olive oil

For the sauce:

- 2 tablespoons low-sodium tamari or soy sauce
- 1 tablespoon rice vinegar
- 1 teaspoon sesame oil
- ½ teaspoon turmeric
- ¼ teaspoon black pepper
- 1 teaspoon honey or maple syrup (optional)

Instructions:

1. Press tofu to remove excess water, then cube.
2. Heat 1 tablespoon olive oil in a wok or large skillet over medium-high heat.
3. Add tofu and cook until golden, about 5 minutes. Remove and set aside.

4. Add remaining oil to the pan.
5. Stir-fry garlic and ginger for 30 seconds.
6. Add vegetables and stir-fry until crisp-tender, 5-7 minutes.
7. Whisk together all sauce ingredients.
8. Return tofu to the pan, add sauce, and toss to coat.
9. Cook for 1-2 more minutes until sauce thickens slightly.

10. Quinoa and Black Bean Stuffed Bell Peppers

Servings: 2
Calories: Approximately 290 calories per serving

Ingredients:

- 2 bell peppers (any color), halved and seeds removed
- ½ cup cooked quinoa
- ½ cup cooked black beans, rinsed and drained
- ¼ cup corn kernels
- 2 tablespoons red onion, diced
- 2 tablespoons cilantro, chopped
- 1 small tomato, diced
- 1 clove garlic, minced
- ½ teaspoon ground cumin
- ¼ teaspoon smoked paprika
- 1 tablespoon olive oil
- 1 tablespoon lime juice
- ¼ cup avocado, diced
- 2 tablespoons pumpkin seeds
- Salt and pepper to taste

Instructions:

1. Preheat oven to 375°F (190°C).
2. Place bell pepper halves cut-side up on a baking sheet.
3. In a bowl, combine quinoa, black beans, corn, red onion, cilantro, tomato, and garlic.
4. Season with cumin, paprika, olive oil, lime juice, salt, and pepper.
5. Stuff mixture into bell pepper halves.
6. Cover with foil and bake for 20 minutes.
7. Remove foil and bake for another 10 minutes.
8. Top with diced avocado and pumpkin seeds before serving.

Dinner - 10 Anti-Inflammatory Mediterranean & Blue Zone Inspired Recipes

Recipes With Chicken Or Fish

1. Mediterranean Herb-Crusted Salmon with Quinoa Pilaf

Servings: 4
Calories per serving: 410

Ingredients:

- 4 salmon fillets (5 oz each)
- 2 tbsp olive oil
- 2 cloves garlic, minced
- 1 tbsp fresh herbs (rosemary, thyme, parsley), chopped
- 1 cup quinoa, rinsed

- 2 cups vegetable broth
- 1 cup cherry tomatoes, halved
- 1 cup kale, chopped
- ¼ cup walnuts, chopped
- 1 lemon, juiced and zested

Instructions:

1. Preheat oven to 400°F.
2. In a bowl, mix olive oil, garlic, herbs, lemon zest, salt, and pepper.
3. Brush salmon with herb mixture and bake for 12-15 minutes.
4. Meanwhile, cook quinoa in vegetable broth until fluffy (about 15 minutes).
5. Fold in tomatoes, kale, walnuts, and lemon juice to the quinoa.
6. Serve salmon over quinoa pilaf.

2. Turmeric-Ginger Chicken with Sweet Potato Mash

Servings: 4
Calories per serving: 385

Ingredients:

- 1.5 lbs chicken breast
- 2 tbsp olive oil
- 2 tsp turmeric powder
- 1 inch fresh ginger, grated
- 3 cloves garlic, minced
- 4 medium sweet potatoes, peeled and cubed
- 2 tbsp Greek yogurt

- 2 cups spinach
- ¼ cup almonds, sliced
- Fresh herbs for garnish

Instructions:

1. Marinate chicken in olive oil, turmeric, ginger, garlic, salt, and pepper for 30 minutes.
2. Boil sweet potatoes until tender, then mash with Greek yogurt.
3. Grill or bake chicken until internal temperature reaches 165°F.
4. Sauté spinach in olive oil until wilted.
5. Serve chicken over sweet potato mash with spinach and garnish with almonds.

3. Asian-Inspired Trout Bowl with Edamame and Broccoli

Servings: 4
Calories per serving: 395

Ingredients:

- 4 trout fillets (5 oz each)
- 2 tbsp olive oil
- 3 tbsp reduced-sodium soy sauce or tamari
- 1 tbsp ginger, grated
- 2 cloves garlic, minced
- 1 cup brown rice
- 2 cups broccoli florets
- 1 cup edamame, shelled
- 1 avocado, sliced

- 2 tbsp sesame seeds
- Green tea for poaching (optional)

Instructions:

1. Cook rice according to package instructions.
2. Steam broccoli and edamame until tender-crisp.
3. In a large skillet, heat olive oil. Cook trout fillets skin-side down for 3-4 minutes.
4. Flip and cook for another 2-3 minutes until done.
5. Make sauce with soy sauce, ginger, and garlic.
6. Serve fish over rice with vegetables, drizzle with sauce, and top with avocado and sesame seeds.

4. Mackerel with Mediterranean Vegetable Medley

Servings: 4
Calories per serving: 425

Ingredients:

- 4 mackerel fillets (5 oz each)
- 2 tbsp olive oil
- 2 cloves garlic, sliced
- 1 cup cherry tomatoes
- 1 cup bell peppers, sliced
- 1 cup zucchini, diced
- ½ cup Kalamata olives
- 1 cup farro, cooked
- ¼ cup pine nuts, toasted
- Fresh herbs (basil, oregano)
- 1 lemon, juiced

Instructions:

1. Cook farro according to package instructions.
2. Heat olive oil in a large skillet. Add vegetables and garlic, sauté until tender.
3. In another pan, cook mackerel fillets 3-4 minutes per side.
4. Toss cooked vegetables with farro, herbs, and lemon juice.
5. Serve mackerel over vegetable-farro mixture, topped with pine nuts.

5. Baked Herbed Chicken with Mushroom and Lentil Stew

Servings: 4
Calories per serving: 405

Ingredients:

- 4 chicken thighs, bone-in, skin removed
- 2 tbsp olive oil
- 2 cups mixed mushrooms, sliced
- 1 cup green lentils, rinsed
- 4 cups low-sodium chicken broth
- 2 carrots, diced
- 2 cloves garlic, minced
- 1 tbsp fresh thyme
- 1 tbsp turmeric
- 1 bay leaf
- 2 cups spinach

Instructions:

1. Preheat oven to 375°F.
2. Season chicken with herbs, salt and pepper. Bake for 30-35 minutes.
3. Meanwhile, heat olive oil in a pot, sauté mushrooms until browned.
4. Add garlic, carrots, lentils, turmeric, thyme, bay leaf, and broth.
5. Simmer for 25-30 minutes until lentils are tender.
6. Stir in spinach just before serving.
7. Serve chicken alongside lentil stew.

Vegetarian/Vegan Recipes

6. Tofu and Vegetable Stir-Fry with Ginger-Turmeric Sauce (Vegan)

Servings: 4
Calories per serving: 350

Ingredients:

- 14 oz extra-firm tofu, pressed and cubed
- 2 tbsp olive oil
- 1 tbsp sesame oil
- 2 cups broccoli florets
- 1 cup bell peppers, sliced
- 1 cup Swiss chard, chopped
- 1 cup edamame, shelled
- 2 cloves garlic, minced
- 1 tbsp ginger, grated
- 1 tbsp turmeric, fresh or powder

- 3 tbsp reduced-sodium soy sauce or tamari
- 1 cup cooked brown rice or quinoa
- 2 tbsp hemp seeds

Instructions:

1. Press and drain tofu for 30 minutes, then cube.
2. Heat olive oil in a wok. Add tofu and cook until golden on all sides.
3. Add vegetables and stir-fry until tender-crisp.
4. Mix sesame oil, garlic, ginger, turmeric, and soy sauce in a small bowl.
5. Pour sauce over stir-fry and toss to coat.
6. Serve over rice or quinoa, topped with hemp seeds.

7. Mediterranean Stuffed Sweet Potatoes (Vegetarian)

Servings: 4
Calories per serving: 380

Ingredients:

- 4 medium sweet potatoes
- 2 tbsp olive oil
- 1 cup chickpeas, drained and rinsed
- 1 cup cherry tomatoes, halved
- ½ cup Kalamata olives, pitted and chopped
- 2 cups spinach, chopped
- 2 cloves garlic, minced
- ½ cup feta cheese (or vegan alternative)
- ¼ cup walnuts, chopped
- 2 tbsp fresh parsley, chopped
- 1 lemon, juiced

Instructions:

1. Preheat oven to 400°F. Poke sweet potatoes with a fork and bake for 45-60 minutes.
2. Heat olive oil in a pan, add garlic and chickpeas. Cook until lightly crisp.
3. Add spinach and cook until wilted.
4. Mix in tomatoes, olives, and lemon juice.
5. Cut open baked sweet potatoes and stuff with the chickpea mixture.
6. Top with feta cheese and walnuts, garnish with parsley.

8. Quinoa Buddha Bowl with Turmeric Tahini Dressing (Vegan)

Servings: 4
Calories per serving: 420

Ingredients:

- 1 cup quinoa, rinsed
- 2 cups mixed greens (kale, arugula)
- 1 cup roasted sweet potato chunks
- 1 cup roasted brussels sprouts
- 1 cup chickpeas, drained and rinsed
- 1 avocado, sliced
- ¼ cup pomegranate seeds
- ¼ cup pumpkin seeds

For the dressing:

- 3 tbsp tahini
- 1 lemon, juiced

- 1 tsp turmeric
- 1 clove garlic, minced
- 1 tsp honey or maple syrup
- Water to thin

Instructions:

1. Cook quinoa according to package instructions.
2. Roast sweet potato chunks and brussels sprouts with olive oil at 400°F for 25 minutes.
3. Make dressing by whisking all dressing ingredients together.
4. Assemble bowls: quinoa, greens, roasted vegetables, chickpeas, and avocado.
5. Drizzle with dressing and top with pomegranate seeds and pumpkin seeds.

9. Mushroom and Lentil Bolognese with Zucchini Noodles (Vegan)

Servings: 4
Calories per serving: 310

Ingredients:

- 2 cups mixed mushrooms, finely chopped
- 1 cup brown lentils, cooked
- 2 tbsp olive oil
- 3 cloves garlic, minced
- 1 cup cherry tomatoes
- 2 cups tomato sauce
- 1 tbsp Italian herbs
- 1 tsp turmeric

- 4 medium zucchinis, spiralized
- ¼ cup nutritional yeast or vegan parmesan
- Fresh basil for garnish

Instructions:

1. Heat olive oil in a large pan. Add mushrooms and cook until browned.
2. Add garlic, cherry tomatoes, and herbs. Cook for 2-3 minutes.
3. Stir in cooked lentils and tomato sauce. Simmer for 10-15 minutes.
4. Meanwhile, lightly sauté zucchini noodles in a separate pan for 2-3 minutes.
5. Serve sauce over zucchini noodles, topped with nutritional yeast and fresh basil.

10. Cauliflower and Chickpea Coconut Curry (Vegan)

Servings: 4
Calories per serving: 370

Ingredients:

- 1 head cauliflower, cut into florets
- 2 cups chickpeas, drained and rinsed
- 1 can (14 oz) coconut milk
- 2 tbsp olive oil
- 1 onion, diced
- 3 cloves garlic, minced
- 1 tbsp ginger, grated
- 2 tsp turmeric
- 1 tsp cumin

- 1 tsp coriander
- 1 cup spinach
- ¼ cup fresh cilantro, chopped
- 1 cup cooked brown rice or quinoa
- ¼ cup toasted almonds

Instructions:

1. Heat olive oil in a large pot. Add onion, garlic, and ginger. Sauté until fragrant.
2. Add spices and cook for 1 minute.
3. Add cauliflower florets and chickpeas, stir to coat with spices.
4. Pour in coconut milk and simmer for 15-20 minutes until cauliflower is tender.
5. Stir in spinach and cook until wilted.
6. Serve over brown rice or quinoa, garnished with cilantro and toasted almonds.

Each recipe incorporates multiple anti-inflammatory ingredients and provides a balanced meal. Feel free to adjust portions or ingredients based on personal preferences or dietary needs!

Conclusion

Fundamentally, this book has explored the intricate ways that inflammation can affect your body, from the gut to the immune system, and how anti-inflammatory superfoods are your solutions to restoring balance. This book has emphasized the benefits of the Mediterranean style diet, which offers a delicious, sustainable approach to eating that supports longevity and vitality. It has also explored how lifestyle modifications, like regular exercise and mindfulness, enhance the positive effects of dietary changes, establishing a holistic path to wellness.

The main takeaway here is clear: **Integrating anti-inflammatory foods into your daily meals can revolutionize your health.** By understanding your body's nutritional needs and embracing a balanced diet, you can significantly reduce inflammation and improve your overall well-being. This book has offered you a blueprint for incorporating these principles into your life, combining the power of food with lifestyle practices to create a harmonious approach to health.

But knowing is just the beginning. It is time to take action. Start small; perhaps try adding a handful of berries to your breakfast or swapping out refined grains for sprouted or whole-grain breads and pastas in your meals. Gradually introduce Mediterranean eating habits, like enjoying more plant-based meals or using olive oil as your cooking staple. These small changes can make a big difference over time. The years of indulging in the standard American diet will not be undone overnight, but you can look forward to feeling better and having more energy in the years to come.

Commitment and consistency are central. Adopting an anti-inflammatory lifestyle is not about quick fixes, but rather, it is about making lasting changes that bring about sustainable health improvements. Be patient with yourself and know that gradual change leads to lasting results. Set personal health goals and celebrate the small victories. Each step forward is a win. Surround yourself with supportive people—whether it is friends, family, or a community group—who encourage your progress and hold you accountable. Their support can make a significant difference, particularly when challenges arise.

Speaking of challenges, it is very normal to encounter them. Life gets busy, social pressures arise, and sometimes, the people around you might not understand your choices. Remember, perseverance is critical. Plan your meals ahead of time to avoid last-minute temptations. If you feel comfortable sharing, communicate your dietary goals with friends and family so they can support you. And when skepticism arises, share your experience with confidence and empathy. This book has provided you with the knowledge and resources to overcome these hurdles.

Now more than ever is the time to take immediate steps toward enhancing your health. Explore the recipes provided in this book, experiment with new foods, and embrace new lifestyle practices. Commit to your health journey with enthusiasm and determination.

I believe in you. Your commitment to learning and improving your health is inspiring. Continue exploring and expanding your knowledge on this topic. There is always more to learn, and every bit of knowledge brings you closer to optimal health. Your future is bright and filled with potential. Embrace it with hope and empowerment. Here's to a healthier, happier you!

Your Review Matters

Dear Reader, before we part I would ask you one favor. Please take 2 minutes to write a review and give your honest opinion.

Your feedback is invaluable to others who are struggling with chronic inflammation and searching for practical, sustainable solutions. By sharing your experience, you can help someone else find their path to better health.

What You Might Include in Your Review

- Did you try any of the recipes? Which ones became your favorites?
- Have you noticed any improvements in your health or energy levels since implementing the anti-inflammatory strategies?
- Which of the top 65 superfoods have you incorporated most regularly into your diet?
- Did you find the information about gut health and inflammation enlightening?

Like many readers, you may have tried various approaches before finding this book. Your unique perspective on how this approach compares to others could be especially helpful.

Scan the QR code to go the review page.

Thank You.

References

Ajmera, Rachael. 2024. "6 benefits of flaxseed oil — plus how to use it." *Healthline*. https://www.healthline.com/nutrition/flaxseed-oil-benefits.

Aldeborgh, Alex. 2024. "Creamy banana avocado smoothie with spinach." *Daisybeet*. https://www.daisybeet.com/creamy-banana-avocado-smoothie-with-spinach/.

American Heart Association. 2025. "American Heart Association recommendations for physical activity in adults and kids." https://www.heart.org/en/healthy-living/fitness/fitness-basics/aha-recs-for-physical-activity-in-adults.

American Heart Association. 2025. "The benefits of beans and legumes." https://www.heart.org/en/healthy-living/healthy-eating/eat-smart/nutri tion-basics/the-benefits-of-beans-and-legumes.

Ashique, Sumel, et al. 2024. "Blueberries in focus: Exploring the phytochemical potentials and therapeutic applications." *Journal of Agriculture and Food Research 18*. https://doi.org/10.1016/j.jafr.2024.101300.

Belkaid, Yasmine, and Timothy Hand. 2015. "Role of microbiota in immunity and inflammation." *Cell 157* (1): 121-141. https://pmc.ncbi.nlm.nih.gov/arti cles/PMC4056765/.

Bell, Simon. n.d. "SMART goals." *Mind Tools*. https://www.mindtools.com/a4wo118/smart-goals.

Bemark, Mats et al. 2024. "Gut-associated lymphoid tissue: A microbiota-driven hub of B cell immunity." *Trends Immunol 45* (3): 211-233. https://pmc.ncbi.nlm.nih.gov/articles/PMC11227984/.

Bjarnadottir, Adda. 2023. "Tomatoes 101: Nutrition facts and health benefits. *Healthline*. https://www.healthline.com/nutrition/foods/tomatoes. *Mediterranean Diet: 8 Scientific Benefits, According to New* ... https://www.healthline.com/health-news/8-ways-the-mediterranean-diet-can-help-you-live-a-longer-and-healthier-life

Blackburn, Kellie Bramlet. 2018. "What happens when you overeat? *The University of Texas MD Anderson Cancer Center*. https://www.mdanderson.org/publica tions/focused-on-health/What-happens-when-you-overeat. h23Z1592202.html.

Cherry, Kendra. 2024. "Self efficacy and why believing in yourself matters." *Verywell Mind*. https://www.verywellmind.com/what-is-self-efficacy-2795954.

Cleveland Clinic. n.d. "Leaky gut syndrome." https://my.clevelandclinic.org/health/diseases/22724-leaky-gut-syndrome.

Continental Hospitals Editorial Team. 2023. "From skin to gut: How junk food affects your body." *Continental Hospitals.* https://continentalhospitals.com/blog/from-skin-to-gut-how-junk-food-affects-your-body/#.

Dominguez, Ligia J, et al. 2024. "Mediterranean diet and spirituality/religion: eating with meaning." *Aging Clinical and Experimental Research 36* (1): 223. https://pubmed.ncbi.nlm.nih.gov/39560850/.

Dryfo. n.d. "The power of herbs and spices in Mediterranean cuisine: Flavour and health benefits." https://dryfo.com/blog-en/articles/the-power-of-herbs-and-spices-in-mediterranean-cuisine-flavor-and-health-benefits/.

Ebrahimi, Peyman, et al. 2023. "Chlorophylls as natural bioactive compounds existing in food by-products: A critical review." *Plants 12* (7): 1533. https://pmc.ncbi.nlm.nih.gov/articles/PMC10096697/.

Furman, David et al. 2019. "Chronic inflammation in the etiology of disease across the life span." *Nature Medicine 25*: 1822-1832. https://www.nature.com/articles/s41591-019-0675-0.

Han, Rui-Min, Jian-Ping Zhang, and Leif H Skibsted. 2012. "Reaction dynamics of flavonoids and carotenoids as antioxidants." *Molecules 17* (2): 2140-2160. https://pmc.ncbi.nlm.nih.gov/articles/PMC6268464/

Harvard Health Publishing. 2024. "How sleep deprivation can cause inflammation." https://www.health.harvard.edu/healthbeat/how-sleep-deprivation-can-cause-inflammation.

Healthdirect. 2023. "Drinking water and your health." https://www.healthdirect.gov.au/drinking-water-and-your-health.

Healthdirect. n.d. "Vitamin A and your health." https://www.healthdirect.gov.au/vitamin-a-and-your-health.

Higdon, Jane V, et al. 2007. "Cruciferous vegetables and human cancer risk: Epidemiologic evidence and mechanistic bias." *Pharmacol Res. 55* (3): 224-236. https://pmc.ncbi.nlm.nih.gov/articles/PMC2737735/.

Hrncir, Tomas. 2022. "Gut microbiota dysbiosis: Triggers, consequences, diagnostic and therapeutic options." *Microorganisms 10* (3): 578. https://pmc.ncbi.nlm.nih.gov/articles/PMC8954387/.

Huang, Zhi, Aaron H Rose, and Peter R Hoffmann. 2012. "The role of selenium in inflammation and immunity: From molecular mechanisms to therapeutic opportunities." *Antioxid Redox Signal 16* (7): 705-743. https://pmc.ncbi.nlm.nih.gov/articles/PMC3277928/.

Indulge. n.d. "Discovering healthy Asian dish options for every palate." https://indulge-food.ch/healthy-asian-dish/.

Jennings, Kerri-Ann. 2023. "7 reasons to eat more citrus fruits." *Healthline.* https://www.healthline.com/nutrition/citrus-fruit-benefits.

John Hopkins Medicine. n.d. "Digestive diagnostic procedures." https://www.hopkinsmedicine.org/health/treatment-tests-and-therapies/digestive-diagnostic-procedures. *Cruciferous Vegetables | Linus Pauling Institute* https://lpi.oregonstate.edu/mic/food-beverages/cruciferous-vegetables

Kalt, Wilhelmina, et al. 2019. "Recent research on the health benefits of blueberries and their anthocyanins." *Advanced Nutrition 11* (2): 224-236. https://pmc.ncbi.nlm.nih.gov/articles/PMC7442370. *Nutrition and Immunity* https://nutritionsource.hsph.harvard.edu/nutrition-and-immunity/

Kasapis, Christos, and Paul D. Thompson. 2005. "The effects of physical activity on serum c-reactive protein and inflammatory markers: A systematic review." *Journal of the American College of Cardiology 45* (10): 1563-1569. https://www.jacc.org/doi/10.1016/j.jacc.2004.12.077.

Kitscha, Phoebe. 2021. "Inflammation: What is it, and how does it affect the heart?" *British Heart Foundation.* https://www.bhf.org.uk/informationsupport/heart-matters-magazine/research/what-is-inflammation.

Kubala, Jillian, and Kris Gunnars. 2024. "8 evidence-based health benefits of quinoa." *Healthline.* https://www.healthline.com/nutrition/8-health-benefits-quinoa.

Kubala, Jillian. 2025. "A guide to essential amino acids and your health." *Healthline.* https://www.healthline.com/nutrition/essential-amino-acids.

Kumar, Ashwani, et al. 2023. "Major phytochemicals: Recent advances in health benefits and extraction method." *Molecules 28* (2): 887. https://pmc.ncbi.nlm.nih.gov/articles/PMC9862941/.

Lakeside Leisure Centre. 2024. "World heart day: The power of exercise for a healthy heart." https://www.lakesideleisure.com.au/news/world-heart-day-the-power-of-exercise-for-a-health.

LeWine, Howard E. 2024. "Foods that fight inflammation." *Harvard Health Publishing.* https://www.health.harvard.edu/staying-healthy/foods-that-fight-inflammation.

LeWine, Howard E. 2024. "Understanding the stress response." *Harvard Health Publishing.* https://www.health.harvard.edu/staying-healthy/understanding-the-stress-response.

Lewis, Sarah. 2024. "Prebiotics vs. probiotics for gut health." *Healthline.* https://www.healthline.com/nutrition/probiotics-and-prebiotics.

Lobo, V. et al. 2010. "Free radicals, antioxidants and functional foods: Impact on human health." *Pharmacogn Rev. 4* (8): 118-126. https://pmc.ncbi.nlm.nih.gov/articles/PMC3249911/.

Mayo Clinic Staff. 2024. "Nutrition and healthy eating." https://www.mayoclinic.org/healthy-lifestyle/nutrition-and-healthy-eating/in-depth/fiber/art-20043983.

National Institutes of Health. n.d. "Your digestive system & how it works." https://www.niddk.nih.gov/health-information/digestive-diseases/digestive-system-how-it-works.

Nunez, Kirsten. 2020. "The benefits of guided imagery and how to do it." *Healthline.* https://www.healthline.com/health/guided-imagery.

Nelson, Joseph B. 2017. "Mindful eating: The art of presence while you eat."

Diabetes Spectrum 30 (3): 171-174. https://pmc.ncbi.nlm.nih.gov/articles/PMC5556586/

Oldways Whole Grains Council. n.d. "What is a whole grain?" https://wholegrainscouncil.org/what-whole-grain.

Pacheco, Danielle, and Anis Rehman. 2024. "Bedroom environment: What elements are important?" https://www.sleepfoundation.org/bedroom-environment.

Pahwa, Roma, Amandeep Goyal, and Ishwarlal Jialal. 2023. "Chronic inflammation." *National Library of Medicine.* https://www.ncbi.nlm.nih.gov/books/NBK493173/. *Gut-associated lymphoid tissue: a microbiota-driven hub of ...* https://www.cell.com/trends/immunology/fulltext/S1471-4906(24)00006-1

Peng, Ying, et al. 2021. "Anti-inflammatory effects of curcumin in the inflammatory diseases: Status, limitations and countermeasures." *Drug Design, Development and Theory 15*: 4503-4525. https://pmc.ncbi.nlm.nih.gov/articles/PMC8572027/.

Philpott, Jenna. 2023. "The healthy eats: How olive oil fits into a nutrient-rich diet." *News-Medical.Net.* https://www.news-medical.net/health/The-Healthy-Fats-How-Olive-Oil-Fits-into-a-Nutrient-Rich-Diet.aspx.

Robinson, Lawrence, Jeanne Segal, and Melinda Smith. 2025. "Relaxation techniques for stress relief." *HelpGuide.org.* https://www.helpguide.org/mental-health/stress/relaxation-techniques-for-stress-relief.

Schervish, Lori. 2018. "Food serving sizes: A visual guide." *EatingWell.* https://www.eatingwell.com/article/290916/food-serving-sizes-a-visual-guide/.

Sethi, Saurabh. 2023. "Malabsorption syndrome." *Healthline.* https://www.healthline.com/health/malabsorption.

Sharifi-Rad, Javad, et al. 2020. "Turmeric and its major compound curcumin on health: Bioactive effects and safety profiles for food, pharmaceutical, biotechnological and medicinal applications." *Frontiers in Pharmacology 11*: 01021. https://pmc.ncbi.nlm.nih.gov/articles/PMC7522354/.

Shin, Yoonhwa, et al. 2023. "Roles of short-chain fatty acids in inflammatory bowel disease." *Nutrients 15* (20): 4466. https://pmc.ncbi.nlm.nih.gov/articles/PMC10609902/.

SHN Staff. 2022. "Sugar crash effects and how to fix them." *Sanford Health.* https://news.sanfordhealth.org/healthy-living/sugar-crash-effects/.

Spritzler, Franziska. 2023. "Salmon nutrition and health benefits." *Healthline.* https://www.healthline.com/nutrition/salmon-nutrition-and-health-benefits#1.

The Nutrition Source. n.d. "Omega-3 fatty acids: An essential contribution." *Harvard T.H. Chan.* https://nutritionsource.hsph.harvard.edu/what-should-you-eat/fats-and-cholesterol/types-of-fat/omega-3-fats/.

U.S. Centers for Disease Control and Prevention. n.d. "About folic acid." https://www.cdc.gov/folic-acid/about/index.html.

Verdu, Elena F, David Armstrong and Joseph A Murray. 2009. "Between Celiac disease and Irritable Bowel Syndrome; The "no man's land" of gluten sensitivity." *American Journal of Gastroenterology 104* (6): 1587-1594. https://pmc.ncbi.nlm.nih.gov/articles/PMC3480312/.

Wartenberg, Lisa. 2023. "7 benefits of drinking lemon-ginger tea before bed." *Healthline.* https://www.healthline.com/nutrition/lemon-ginger-tea-before-bed#constipation.

Yaseen, Kinanah. 2024. "Overview of systemic rheumatic diseases." *MSD Manual.* https://www.msdmanuals.com/home/bone-joint-and-muscle-disorders/systemic-rheumatic-diseases/overview-of-systemic-rheumatic-diseases.

YouFit. 2025. "Bust through that plateau & reignite your fitness journey." https://youfit.com/blog/bust-through-that-plateau-reignite-your-fitness-journey/

El Nabli, Jasmine MS, RDN "Top 10 Anti-inflammatory Fighting Foods" https://parentishealth.com/top-10-anti-inflammatory-fighting-foods/